HEALING THROUGH ILLNESS, LIVING THROUGH DYING

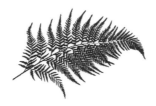

Guidance and Rituals for Patients, Families, and Friends

BY CANDICE C. COURTNEY

Foreword by Kenneth J. Doka, Ph.D.

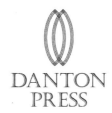

DANTON
PRESS

Healing Through Illness, Living Through Dying:
Guidance and Rituals for Patients, Families, and Friends
Copyright © 2012 Candice C. Courtney
ISBN 978-0-9850522-2-5

Danton Press
7904 Chaparral Road #A110-428
Scottsdale, AZ 85250
(480) 664-7790
www.DantonPress.com
info@DantonPress.com

Disclaimer
This book includes information from many sources and from personal experiences. It is published for general reference and is not intended to be a substitute for medical, legal, or financial advice. The publisher and author shall not be liable for any special, consequential, or exemplary damages resulting, in whole or in part, from the reader's use of, or reliance on, the information contained in this book. The author and publisher bear no responsibility for the persistence or accuracy of URLs for external or third-party Internet web sites referred to in this publication and do not guarantee that any content on such web sites will remain accurate or appropriate.

Cover and Book Design by Sherry Wachter
Author Photographs by Andy Rodriguez Photography

Editorial and Production Services
Maureen Michelson, NewSage Press

Printed in the United States

Library of Congress Control Number: 2012931960

DEDICATION

To Tony
because we loved
all the way through

Contents

Foreword

*A*rnold Van Gennep, a French ethnologist, once described rituals as liminal. The word has considerable power. This means that rituals exist in that transitional space between consciousness and unconsciousness. When we participate in a ritual, we obviously are doing this in a way that is conscious and available to us. Yet, often something in the ritual may touch us unconsciously—in a way less accessible to the mind. Think, for example, of being at a wedding and becoming inexplicably tearful, or getting goose bumps at patriotic rituals. In each of these events, we responded at both a conscious and unconscious level.

I define ritual as investing an act with meaning. For example, I am a Lutheran clergyman and communion is usually an important aspect of our Worship Ritual. In communion we partake of bread and wine. At a restaurant, the waiter brings bread to the table, and I might order a glass of wine. The same elements are present, but this act is not communion. Yet, invest the same elements of bread and wine with a deeper meaning, and one is involved in a sacred ritual.

Since rituals are meaningful acts that exist in the liminal space between consciousness and unconsciousness, they have power. Even before history, there was ritual. The tombs of prehistoric peoples bear witness to the elaborate rites that accompanied death even before we had the ability to document those rites.

Rituals create not only meaning but connection. They engender community. They allow us to do something at a stressful time—bringing a sense of purpose and order to a chaotic time. Rituals remind us of the ways that our beliefs—philosophy or faith—speak to us in a time of crisis.

Candice Courtney's *Healing Through Illness, Living Through Dying: Guidance and Rituals for Patients, Families, and Friends* builds on this power. As Candice faced her husband's final illness, she found ritual to be an important way to cope with the illness and impending loss. Courtney is sensitive to the process of illness. She creates rituals at distinct phases of the illness—at the time of diagnosis, during the chronic period as they live with the disease, in the terminal period as they face death, and the inevitable funeral.

Beyond these powerful options for rituals, Courtney offers additional insights for patients and families as they cope with life-threatening illness. She is sensitive to another aspect of liminality. In the transitional space between life and death, Courtney is sensitive to the possibilities that exist for personal growth, transformation, and the development of deeper relationships with others.

Patients, families, and friends will find both comfort and wisdom in this book. Therapists, counselors, clergy, and health professionals will find a treasure trove of useful ideas as they work with patients and families coping with life-threatening illness and loss. *Healing Through Illness, Living Through Dying* illustrates a core concept of her journey—that even in painful experiences, there are opportunities to share and to grow.

— KENNETH J. DOKA, PH.D.
Professor, The College of New Rochelle
Senior Consultant, The Hospice Foundation of America

Introduction

This is a book about healing, and loving, and living. It is also a book about facing serious illness. Due to some astonishing medical advances, many patients today are cured of their disease. Equally amazing is that some individuals are healed by their disease. Confronting a life-threatening illness can open eyes and hearts in such a way that something deep within opens to healing. Old emotional wounds are salved, counter-productive attitudes shed, and the frantic pace of life slowed. As part of the same process, generosity of spirit, love, appreciation, and deeper meaning become luminous.

The healing of body and psyche can postpone death, sometimes for months, sometimes for years, but not forever. We will all die one day. The rituals in this book can help you heal through illness, and live more fully through all of life's passages; even life's last, most difficult, and perhaps, most meaningful passage.

After being diagnosed with a malignant brain tumor, my husband, Tony, would periodically say, "I don't know how to prepare for death."

I would answer, "The only thing I know to do to prepare for it is to live as fully and as well as one can until then."

This was not a wrong answer, but it was decidedly incomplete. I quickly learned how to navigate through the medical world so Tony could have every possible chance at being one of the rare individuals who survived his form of brain tumor. It was more difficult, though, to understand how best to help him navigate the personal passages on our journey.

Together, we moved through the twenty-two months following his diagnosis the best we knew how. Sometimes we stumbled through reasonably well, and there were times we moved with strength and grace. However, some important things were put off, avoided, or simply went unnoticed.

Nobody does everything perfectly, in sickness or in health. I now know there are many ways to prepare for death, to fight for more time, and to live as fully as possible until the very end of life. If I had it to do over again, I would have a more complete answer for Tony.

Healing Through Illness, Living Through Dying is the book I wish we'd had to help us better understand our options. I hope it provides you, the reader, with the means to move through your journey with fewer regrets and greater grace.

—CANDICE C. COURTNEY
January 2012

PART ONE

Getting Your Bearings

Chapter 1

Living Fully with a Serious Illness

Diagnosis of a serious illness pushes the world sideways, turns stomachs upside down, and radically rearranges priorities. There is suddenly much to learn about the disease, the various options for treatment, and the problematic side effects of drugs. Overwhelmed with fighting for more life and negotiating for better quality of that life, it is easy to lose sight of the fact that in the midst of all this—there is still a life to be lived.

The rituals in *Healing Through Illness, Living Through Dying* will prompt you to remember what it is that feeds and heals your greater self. You will find suggestions, exercises, and rituals offering perspective, along with a broader sense of the options open to you at any given time. This book is not a to-do list, but a map of places you may want or need to visit.

For some patients, the journey will take them into recovery for many years, while for others the chances of remission are slim. No one ever knows for certain what the future will bring, but an alarming prognosis brings a face-to-face confrontation with great uncertainty. Whether the doctor's prognosis is somber or encouraging, a life-threatening diagnosis causes people to suddenly realize that we—all of us—really are mortal, and death may come sooner than expected.

The threat of death can hang over us like a shadow, but shining a light on it can help release some of the dread and anxiety. If we know what to expect, we may fear it less. If we put our affairs in order, we will release certain burdens. If we see our true priorities, we can more gracefully enter into the fullness of the time that's left us, however long or short it may be.

Lessons Learned from Being Present

I was thirty-five the first time I was a part of someone's death. My Uncle Ray was dying, and I didn't know what to expect, or what was expected of me. I had lost two cousins, two other uncles, and all of my grandparents, but I had not been present with any of them in their dying, and I was glad I hadn't been. Death had seemed so awful until I witnessed it.

Uncle Ray was at home with family in attendance. I don't think any of us had previously been present with someone during the last hours and at the moment of passing. Our instincts guided us fairly well even though we felt helpless and unsure. We did what we could to help Uncle Ray be comfortable, and we told him how much we cared about him.

My Uncle Ray taught me many things about life when I was still new to this world, and it seems most fitting that he taught me, and my family, valuable lessons about death as he was leaving this life. Most importantly, we learned that death doesn't have to be frightening and awful; the act of dying can be simple, profound, and even beautiful. When I later read Elisabeth Kubler-Ross's words, "Being present at a peaceful death is like witnessing a shooting star," I knew exactly what she meant.

When my father died seven years after Uncle Ray, my family was more deeply impacted, but we were less unsure, more comfortable, able to be more present, and so, better able to offer him support.

I mourned the deaths of my favorite uncle and my dad, yet I was most grateful for the lessons learned in their dying when I had to support my husband, Tony, on his journey through the end of life.

Tony's diagnosis demanded much of both of us. It sometimes frightened us, always challenged us, yet it also provoked certain things within us to blossom in some completely unexpected ways. Together, we learned that alongside the uncertainty and sadness there can be growth and healing, humor, and the strength of love.

Notes on Using This Book

This book does not need to be read in any particular order. Part One provides a foundation, then feel free to turn to whichever chapter addresses your immediate needs, or piques your curiosity.

Part Two, "A Map of Patients' Choices," contains rituals to help the patient and caregiver reorient following diagnosis, or at other junctures in their journey. The rituals in Part Two help patients create space for reflection, and invite expression of thoughts and feelings. The chapters on taking care of business and taking care of one's self encourage a clearer understanding of priorities, and offer support in following through. Part Two also includes rituals that can bring deeper meaning, growth, healing, and greater joy into the journey for both patient and caregiver.

Part Three, "A Map for Family and Friends," provides rituals that family and friends can call upon in offering support to the patient following diagnosis, through treatment, and during the final passages of life. The rituals also support family and friends, encouraging them to more gracefully act on their natural impulses. (Some patients might want to look through Part Three and indicate their preferences.) There are also rituals to support family and friends as they move through the first few days following their loss.

Part Four, "Specific Circumstances," addresses particular areas that may be important for certain readers. For example, the chapter on children includes helpful information whether the child is the patient, a family member, or simply visiting. Sometimes, patients near the end of life will have symptoms of dementia, even if that wasn't an issue previously. A familiarity with what is included may prove helpful for you should you want or need the information at some point along your journey.

All online resources listed in this book are also provided on my website, www.healingthroughillness.com.

These rituals are suggestions and ideas. Choose what holds meaning or value for you. As suggested previously, approach it like a map—some places you may want to visit, others you'll drive right past, and one or two might be worth extra effort even if that requires going out of your way, or getting off the beaten path.

CHAPTER 2

When the World Shifts

*I*n March of 1997, my husband was diagnosed with a brain tumor and given only months to live. It felt like the whole world was knocked sideways. Our priorities shifted dramatically, and most of life's ordinary routines were altered or abandoned. It was hard to get our bearings, and difficult to keep our balance in the midst of so many sudden changes. Like most people, we had to figure it out as we went.

Doctors guide patients through the medical steps of addressing the disease, but most patients and caregivers also need some guidance on how to move forward through the other parts of life.

We need help understanding how to focus on life now that life doesn't feel quite our own anymore. We need support in finding ways to express our thoughts and feelings. We may need help demonstrating to others how we are choosing to deal with the circumstance, and how we would like them to interact with us. Ritual can help guide us, help keep us in better balance, and nurture us along the journey.

Uncertainty

The future suddenly becomes an unpredictable place. My husband Tony had bouts of being angry and frustrated that he couldn't plan for a future anymore. One day he said, "I don't know what's going to happen to me. Even if this new treatment works and I live, what kind of shape will I be in?"

Patients' lives, emotions and bodies feel so out of control when stripped of the illusion that they have some control over the future.

Periodically I would remind Tony that the future was no more unpredictable now than it had ever been. The difference was that now we had become all too aware of that fact. We had suffered a loss of innocence.

The truth is that everyone's future is unpredictable; no one truly knows what it will hold. Others, at least for now, are allowed to go on believing that they can plan their future. Yet any one of them could be hit by a truck or by lightning at any moment. The future is not, and never was, an orderly and secure place.

But how do we live without that false, but comfortable, illusion of security? How do we live in uncertainty? An old proverb with a small twist serves as guidance:

Prepare for the worst.
Hope and prepare for the best.
Live in the now.

Living in the Now

Life doesn't stop with a diagnosis of serious illness, but it changes it, intensifies it, and suddenly the present matters more than it did a month ago.

Tony and I found ourselves living much more in the moment— not because of meditation practice or anything Zen or even Timothy Leary, but because each day demanded so much from us. The time before diagnosis seemed strangely foreign, and the future was too uncertain to plan beyond next week's doctor appointments. We had no choice but to live in the moment, and we grew together through that experience daily.

How did we get through it? One appointment at a time. One meal at a time. One MRI at a time. One round of pills at a time. One hug at a time. One walk holding hands at a time. One load of laundry at a time. And we exercised our love and our humor all the time—especially when things were at their worst.

Tony and I both did our best to face it head on, to see his disease as a challenge and an opportunity for growth. This does not mean we didn't feel overwhelmed by it all at times, yet both of us found strengths we didn't know we possessed. We developed as individuals, and as a couple, in whole new areas.

Unexpected Gifts

Surprisingly, healing and growth can happen on many levels because of serious illness. Opening ourselves to the love that is around us, and more openly expressing love to others, is one of those strange but wonderful gifts that serious illness offers us. The disease takes much with one hand, but offers some rare and beautiful privileges with the other hand.

I found that I could handle far more than I would have thought. I also learned a different kind of selflessness that did not feel as if I were diminishing my self.

Tony steadily became more physically dependent on me, but he learned that I honored his independence of spirit no less. And so, his dependence taught him a stronger sense of trust. His vulnerability opened him to give and receive greater love.

Be alert for the gifts that will be offered you on your own journey.

Loss of Control

Most of us feel great discomfort in a state of limbo, particularly one where the thought is, "I may survive this and have a few more years, but still...."

The "when" of death is out of our control, and this can make us feel as if everything is out of our control. This can be felt so acutely we forget that much of the "how" is still within our power. When given time to prepare for death, we have the opportunity to round things out and close the circle of life in a way that can hold meaning for all of those involved. As one woman voiced it, "There is an odd privilege in being given some notice that I may be reaching the end of my life."

Hope and Prepare

Tony wanted to prepare for death. I hoped and believed that if we stayed focused on making it through we would not need to prepare for it. I thought, *If the time comes that we need to give up hope of survival, we can prepare then.* But when we reached that point, there wasn't time to prepare. I now understand that preparing doesn't preclude hope.

Hope for the best, prepare for the worst. Fervently hope. Deeply, desperately, confidently pray for miracles. But also prepare for death's ultimate arrival, which will happen for each and every one of us. No one knows exactly when. Preparing for death can actually help relieve stress, release certain burdens, and help clear the way so that what matters most has room to blossom.

Addressing these needs through ritual, or otherwise, can co-exist with hope. I've heard many stories of those who took care of unfinished business, from writing wills to settling grievances, and then they went into remission and lived for years. Whether it was because of freeing the self of burdens and relieving certain stresses, we cannot know. Preparing for death may not push it away, but looking at it as a real possibility and preparing for it most certainly does not bring it on.

Facing our own death can offer us a different force to live. It is not without despair, but it can offer a more focused present—now things can no longer be put off until next year. We have to ask ourselves, "What do I need to do before my spirit leaves this earth and this body behind? Which things are primary?" And also, "What do I truly want and need today?"

The time left may be shorter than what had previously been anticipated, so what is most important? Is it to visit China, finish a work in progress, or spend time with family? Sometimes, there is a desire for something major, but more often it is the small things in life that suddenly seem more important and fulfilling. Answering some of the following questions can be helpful when trying to sort out a new sense of priorities:

How do you want to make the most of the time you have?

What are your goals?

How do you want to travel this path?

What are the places you want to visit along the way?

If you die, what do you want that to be like?

If you recover, how will your life change?

How can you move forward with open arms, and an open heart?

In addition to making more conscious use of our time, we can use the nearness of death for greater appreciation of the world and all that's in it. Dylan Thomas wrote, "The closer I move to death, the louder the sun blooms." I was often reminded of that line of poetry as I watched sunsets with my dad in his last two months.

Not only does the world shift with a serious diagnosis, but the way we look at the world also shifts. While aspects of this are unsettling, to say the least; there can also be a stronger sense of what truly matters in life, and a renewed sense of appreciation for the lovely and the ordinary.

CHAPTER 3

Understanding Ritual

Ritual can be public and formal like a wedding or the inauguration of a president. It can also be simple and ordinary like shaking hands when introduced to someone. In these, and many other situations, ritual offers a template that helps us know what to do.

When we meet someone new we generally follow the established pattern of exchanging: "How do you do?" "It's nice to meet you." This tiny ritual gives us the half-minute we need to get a sense of the person and to figure out what we want to say next. It provides a structure that supports us as we make that very small transition.

Death is a huge transition, the greatest one since birth. The months or years between diagnosis and death involve many transitions, and so we need many different rituals to help us as we move from the disruption of diagnosis through various ups and downs until we come to the end of life. That time may be only a few months as it was with my dad, or almost two years as it was with my husband, or in some cases, even decades of treatment-free living. Whatever the time frame may be, ritual can support and enrich you throughout your journey.

One way that ritual supports us is through the use of symbols or symbolic action, such as the exchange of rings in a wedding ceremony. When we shake hands, we make a literal and figurative connection with the other person. We regularly use a wide variety of such symbols in our lives without always being aware of them, yet the inherent symbolism usually resonates within us.

Taking off our work clothes and slipping into something more comfortable at the end of the day helps us to feel looser and more relaxed—in part because of the comfy sweats or shorts, but also because we have shed symbols of our work day. It is part practical and part symbolic, as many rituals are. Taking several deep breaths and letting go of work-related problems as we exhale can enhance this small ritual and help us shed even more of the job and its pressures when we change clothes.

Throughout this book there are a number of simple rituals such as this that can easily slip into everyday routines, as well as special occasion rituals that require planning.

How Ritual Serves Us

Serious illness can cause us to feel isolated from the "regular" world, other people, and cut off even from ourselves at times. Ritual can provide us with a sense of connection on a number of levels. Gathering in a circle creates a sense of social connection. Spiritual connections are made through rituals like communion. At its best, ritual brings us into connection with our deepest and truest self.

Ritual offers a way into doing what we instinctively want to do, but may not know if we should, or how to go about it.

Ritual shows us how to gracefully transition into, through, and then out of, new or uncomfortable situations.

Ritual can create a safe space for raw expression of thoughts and feelings. Reflecting upon those thoughts and feelings can help us discern what will create a greater sense of wholeness.

Ritual can help us combat feelings of helplessness through understanding what our options are.

Ritual can help us discover a way of resolving something that troubles us; repairing relationships, finding forgiveness, even reaching into the future.

The following story of a father diagnosed with cancer illustrates a few of the many different needs that can be met through ritual.

In a ritual to express and release anger at the prospect of dying too soon, John chanted and shouted his thoughts and feelings while beating on a drum. Through this he realized that his greatest anger was fueled by grief at not getting to watch his children grow up, and not being able to guide and help them along their path.

In talking about this, John came to see he could still be a part of their development after his death. He wrote letters to each child to be opened at different junctures in their lives; when they turned sixteen and twenty-one years old, when they were choosing a career, when they got married, and when they had their first child. Through this, he was able to fulfill a certain part of parenting he didn't want to lose. John discovered that by envisioning each child at those ages, in some way he did get to "see" them growing up.

The first ritual of simply being able to vent his anger was helpful for John. The second ritual of writing the letters was deeply meaningful in so many ways. Opening those letters will become a ritual for his children, and through this, they will be able to connect with their father over the years and feel his presence at key times in their lives.

Working with Ritual

No ritual is right for everyone, so I offer a range of rituals to suit different needs, different styles. Choose what holds meaning or value for you.

You may find many of the rituals appealing, or only a few. Some may work for you exactly as they are, but with others you may need to reshape the general idea so it feels more comfortable, or better addresses your needs.

If only a small piece of a particular ritual holds meaning for you, take that piece and make it your own. Ritual is most meaningful when it addresses the specific needs of an individual, and in a manner consistent with her or his style and values. Give yourself the creative latitude to do what feels right in altering the rituals so they are a better fit for you.

There is, though, a structure to ritual that needs to be respected. The exact wording of "nice to meet you" can be changed, but the general format is followed: exchanging a few friendly words, making contact, then an open period of conversation followed by something like, "Nice to have met you," or "I hope to see you again" to provide a closing.

The most important part of ritual is what happens in the "empty" spaces—conversations and connections that happen in between. Ritual creates a container for the connections to happen.

Chapter 6, "Gathering with Friends and Family," offers a primer on taking a basic idea and bending it different ways to suit different people.

All of the rituals in this book can be done on your own, though in some cases it may be beneficial to enlist someone to lead, such as a friend, therapist, or clergyperson. If you don't know someone who would serve well, check with a local support group or hospice agency to see if they can offer a recommendation.

The rituals don't need to be done in any particular order, and it may be that a ritual from the first part of the book might be done much later. Rituals can also be repeated at different times.

Ritual Created Through Intent

Almost anything can be made into a ritual through focus of intent, even something as simple and ordinary as breathing.

"I breathe in cleansing and healing energy. As I breathe out, I let go of tensions and toxins."

Inhaling and exhaling not only take on symbolic meaning, but there is also a physical response. The body begins to relax, and mental tensions are reduced. While we cannot as readily perceive the impact of other intents in the ritual, it is likely that these also happen on some level.

Rituals of Gratitude

There are a number of rituals in this book that suggest focusing on gratitude. Expressing gratitude is healing for us, like putting salve on a wound. It invites us to not just count our blessings, but to feel our blessings.

Focusing on gratitude opens the heart and enables connections with our selves and with others. I find it interesting that many traditional prayers begin and end with expressing gratitude to a higher power.

Expressing gratitude is a way of connecting to The Holy, however it is perceived. Gratitude connects us with our own holiness, and it helps us connect with a sense of wholeness. (The word "holy" derives from the word "whole.") In the wake of something painful or difficult, it is healing to connect with a sense of wholeness. Gratitude is a wonderful means to that end.

This book is not an exhaustive listing of rituals that could be done, but I hope you find rituals here that help you. And I hope these ideas provide you with inspiration to create other rituals.

PART TWO

A Map of Patients' Choices

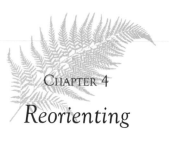

CHAPTER 4

Reorienting

*T*hroughout our lives, there are times when we have to reorient ourselves. Changing jobs, moving to a new home, marrying, or divorcing, all ask that we not only realign our thinking, but relearn our selves and our world in certain ways.

Diagnosis of a life-threatening illness is a far bigger and more difficult turn for everyone involved. Suddenly, patients have to alter the way they think about everything in life: how they work, play, exercise, eat, and sleep. Even their body no longer seems quite the same. Daily routines give way to accommodate doctors' appointments, medical tests, hospital stays, and procedures.

Discomfort, fatigue, fears, and vulnerabilities, all affect how you relate to practically everything. The focus of your conversation shifts. Medical advances become far more riveting than election returns. Fashion trends or the next sporting event may have been important a month ago, but suddenly these things can seem totally trivial.

The mind reels because so much changes so suddenly. In order to find some kind of balance in the midst of this chaos, you will have to reorient or you will remain in a state where everything is swirling around you. Reorienting happens over time as you address large and small aspects of your new circumstances, and learn *your* way to function in a dramatically changed situation. First, though, you must recover your equilibrium.

Regaining Balance

Recovering balance can help us regain some sense of control, and enable us to find our calm center. When we are physically off balance, we steady ourselves by reaching out to hold on to something stable—a railing or another person. When we are mentally or emotionally off balance, we also need to grab hold of something that can steady us. Identify what provides you with emotional stability. Then, find an object to serve as a reminder or touchstone that you can literally hold onto when feeling especially off balance. This symbol might be a smooth stone from your favorite river, or a seashell you found on the beach, rosary beads, or maybe a keepsake from someone you love. Keep this special symbol handy, perhaps in your pocket or by your bedside, and regularly hold it in your hand, or in your mind, to bring you back to your grounded center.

Imbalance and anxiety sometimes become entwined, each making the other worse. If anxiety accompanies your imbalance—as crazy as this may sound—literally hold onto a table or lean against a wall while mentally connecting with what provides a sense of balance. I remember leaning against the refrigerator on a number of occasions and feeling as if it literally held me up.

Dancers are good examples of how to maintain balance when spinning. A dancer "spots" when doing turns, focusing on the same spot with each revolution to prevent dizziness as she spins. You can use this trick, too. Keep coming back to a focus point that you can easily locate. It might be telling yourself repeatedly, "I love my kids, I can get through today." Perhaps, "God's light surrounds me," or "I have the strength to grow and develop through this part of my life."

A yoga pose can be helpful to reestablish stability. Take time to figure out what provides this for you. You may need to experiment a bit to find what works best, and what works may change as your circumstances change. It is possible that the perfect thing might come to you and hold throughout this journey, but not always. When the dancer moves from the rehearsal hall to the stage, she will have to find a different spot to focus on in order to stay oriented. Similarly, our life circumstances keep changing, and we have to do so, too.

Remember, even if we completely lose our balance on occasion, we only fall to the ground. Fanny on the floor, we do recover our balance. And hopefully it helps us recover our sense of humor!

Counterbalance

In the midst of all the upheaval and adjustments of living with a serious illness, it's important to make sure your life doesn't get too far out of balance. It is easy for the disease to take over too much of life. Think about where you might need to add counterbalance. If your days are all too full and busy, schedule time to retreat and slow down for a while, doing little or nothing. If you had a week filled with medical appointments, on the weekend take a drive into the country, breathe fresh air, and enjoy the beauty of nature. If you can't leave town, you could order take-out from a nice restaurant and light candles. Or you might watch a favorite comedy and invite family or friends to share the laughter. Do something that provides a sense of pleasure and camaraderie.

When it feels like there is too much that is too difficult in your day, allow yourself to step outside of it for a moment and think of three things that are easy in your life. If you can, write them down as an extra reminder. This will help counterbalance the overwhelming challenges. It won't make them go away, or even make them less challenging, but it does provide a more balanced perspective on your life. There is always something positive or good, even in the most stressful times—you need only bring your attention to it.

I discovered this on a particularly awful day when, on top of the regular difficulties, my husband and I were faced with additional problems. First, the medical lab notified us that there had been a problem, and we'd have to go back to the hospital to redo Tony's blood draw. We didn't really have an extra hour in our day to take care of this, but it had to be done. Leaving the lab for the second time that day, we went out to our car only to discover that someone had run into it and had mangled the front bumper. The person didn't have the grace or honor to leave a note with contact information. When we got home, we found a note stuck in our door from the landlord saying he was raising our rent. It all seemed like too much, and I wanted to just cave in and crumple in a heap on the kitchen floor. Then it hit me, "I've got to get to the store, we're out of food!" I started to come unglued over this last problem before Tony reminded me that we had gone to the market the day before.

Suddenly, I was relieved and elated, "We don't have to go to the grocery store!" Things suddenly shifted. Breathing a sigh of relief, I relaxed and released some of the tension. "The car repair can wait until we have time to deal with it. And while the rent increase isn't welcomed, we can handle it."

Simply thinking of three things that made life a little easier made a significant change in my attitude. I didn't have to go the market, didn't have to deal with the car right away, and we were fortunate enough that the rent increase wouldn't be a huge burden. We were, I realized, actually quite blessed. "Well, at least we don't have to run to the market!" became a running joke. Humor always helps bring a sense of balance to a situation.

We tend to think of balance in terms of two sides—left or right, dark or light, east or west—but that is two-dimensional thinking and we live in a three-dimensional world. So, in terms of general balance, it is helpful to think of three areas of life. Cameras and telescopes rest on tripods because of the greater stability offered by three legs. What are three touch points you can use to give you the stability you need? For example, it could be medical care, family, and faith, or perhaps promoting a healthier body, socializing with friends, and continuing your artwork. Once you identify three areas of your life that provide a sense of stability, make sure that there is time in your weekly, if not daily, schedule for all three.

If these suggestions seem overwhelming right now, then begin with a simple yet essential practice—three-point breathing. Slowly, take a deep breath in, pause, and let the air rise, allowing it to lift you with it. Then slowly exhale and release tension. Do this three times, or do three sets of three breaths, whenever you need to bring yourself back into balance. If nothing else works, focusing on your breath will help ground you in the moment, and rejuvenate your body with extra oxygen.

Discovering a New Compass

The changes we encounter after diagnosis, recurrence, or even remission, require new directions and new ways to navigate unknown territory. Each person's journey will be different, but there are some things that can help whatever your particular situation involves.

The word orient means "to rise" at its Latin root, and is associated with the sun rising in the east. (This is why the Far East is referred to as "The Orient.") So, if you are reorienting by facing east—both literally and figuratively—you are gaining a sense of your bearings. In essence, orienting one's self is a matter of determining where you are with reference to circumstances or geography.

In both literal and metaphorical terms, the rising sun illuminates the dark, and hence, you are able to see where you are. Facing east is about really seeing the truth. Not only facing the hard truth of changed circumstances, but also about finding your own inner truth. Then you can ask yourself, "What choices will be in alignment with my truest values?"

When seeking a compass to help determine which direction to take, the realm of symbolism can provide questions to help you orient with your truest self:

The East asks, "What do you see as your truth?"

The South asks, "What is your passion?"

The question from the West is, "What to let go of in order to flow a little better?"

North invites you to discover, "What is your fixed point, your North Star?"

The last question is especially important, because your answer helps you know what holds true for you through changes, just as the North Star in the night sky has guided sailors for millennia through changing seas and seasons. What is your North Star? For some, it is a cause to which they are deeply committed, for others their faith, or love of family. It is important that you know where your North Star is in order to stay focused when everything is swirling around you, or pulling you down, or when you feel lost and alone in the midst of a vast, turbulent ocean.

Face these four directions periodically and allow yourself to thoughtfully answer these questions. Don't reach for the familiar response—that may no longer hold true for you. Your answers will not be the same as they would have been a year ago, and they may not be the same next week. As we journey through time and space we must reorient ourselves over and over again, each time anew.

Discerning the Right Path

To begin discovering the road to take in moving forward, write a paragraph or two to describe where you are right now. If you are inclined to write more than that, do so, but it can be as simple as these two examples illustrate:

> *Three weeks ago I was diagnosed with a malignant brain tumor. I'm starting radiation and trying to comprehend the chemotherapy options. It's all swirling around me. Sometimes it seems surreal, and other times so frighteningly real that I forget to breathe.*

Or perhaps:

> *The MRI confirmed that the cancer is in remission. I've hoped and prayed for this, yet as I walked out of the doctor's office, I didn't feel the jubilation I'd expected, not even relief—okay, some sense of relief, but not huge relief. I actually feel kind of disoriented, even a little bit sad at not getting to see Wendy the chemo nurse anymore. It's weird.*

Once you get a good idea of where you honestly are at this point in time, you can better determine what your choices are, and what direction to take. Make a list of options, such as:

Follow my doctor's recommendations for treatment.

Get a second, or third opinion.

Become better informed.

Gather friends and family around.

Go to Disneyland and not think about it for a few days.

Think of all the possible choices you have, then let yourself ponder which direction feels most right for you. Do one small thing to move toward it. Then make a list of the next steps to take. Once you have a plan and are moving forward with it, there is often a sense of relief.

Your Personal Orientation Program

An orientation is generally considered a program or class to introduce us to a new environment, job, or school. A life-threatening illness puts us in a new environment, and our new job becomes educating ourselves about the illness and treatment options. Just like attending a university, there are many lessons to be learned in a variety of classrooms. Life asks each of us to discover what matters most, and then make our choices accordingly. We each have to develop our own orientation program, so to speak, and fortunately, there are many resources and informed people who can help.

For starters, be sure to ask doctors what side effects are likely as a result of your treatment. Also, ask nurses. Since they often spend more time with patients, they generally hear more than doctors about what patients experience in terms of side effects. Nurses are usually a wealth of information for handling common problems related to chemo and radiation treatments.

Seek out patient support groups. Generally, you can learn a lot from listening to other patients, and they may give you a broader sense of what to expect on your journey, as well as provide coping suggestions.

Talking with others who more fully understand certain things you're going through can help you feel more grounded, and less isolated. And because each person is unique, the differences between individuals can be enlightening. Varied circumstances, differences in strengths and weaknesses, can help you see where you are with greater clarity.

Ask an oncology coordinator, hospitalist, or hospital social worker for referrals. Also, check online or in your local phone book for support groups. There are general groups for cancer or heart disease, as well as disease-specific groups, such as leukemia, breast cancer, hepatitis C, AIDS, and ALS, among others.

You may have to look around and try different groups to find one that is right for you. Whether the support group is online or in person, it can be enormously helpful. (See "Resources" for more suggestions.)

Another important source of support is palliative care, which many hospitals now offer, though sometimes you need to specifically request it.

For a cancer patient, the oncologist is focused on treating your cancer, but the palliative care team is focused on improving the quality of your life while undergoing treatment. Palliative care can help alleviate certain symptoms, side effects of drugs, as well as pain and stress resulting from the disease. Any patient with a serious illness, at any stage, can benefit from working with a palliative care team.

This team includes doctors, nurses, social workers, and other specialists, who take time with patients and their families to help them better understand treatment options. The team works with your other doctors to provide an extra layer of support, and works with you to see that you get the best possible treatment and care for your condition. A fact sheet on palliative care states, "A number of studies in recent years have shown that patients who have their symptoms controlled, and are able to communicate their emotional needs, have a better experience with their medical care. Their quality of life and physical symptoms improve."

Because the team members also address many of the psychosocial and spiritual aspects of life affected by diagnosis, they can help you in reorienting by providing a stronger framework of support.

Orienting one's self is about making necessary adjustments, figuring out where you are, and which way to move next. At its root, and deepest meaning, to orient means "to rise." Understanding your self and what is important to you, will enable you in rising to meet the challenges before you. You will meet some of them with astonishing strength and grace, and others not quite so well. Rise to meet each challenge the best you can at that moment, be gentle with yourself, try not to judge, and keep breathing through it all.

Most importantly, stay connected with your truth as best you can, for this will serve as your compass, and this book provides a map.

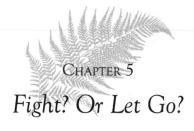

CHAPTER 5

Fight? Or Let Go?

*I*nitial diagnosis of serious illness often prompts a response of, "Let's fight this. I want more life, more time." In many situations, seeking a cure or an extension of life is obviously the right choice. Sometimes, the pros and cons of treatment discomfort must be weighed against potential length of time and the quality of that life.

I know of a number of cases where patients have survived months, years, and even decades beyond what doctors anticipated. Yet, even those who fully recover from a critical injury or life-threatening disease will someday arrive at the moment of letting go. At some point in time, each one of us will let go of the fight for survival. It may happen only seconds before we take our last breath, or there may be a period of letting go in stages over many months or years. I have witnessed people, animals, and even plants reaching toward life as long as possible, and then in grace, letting go. The survival instinct is powerful in all living things, and the wisdom and grace of knowing when to let go is no less awe-inspiring.

Fighting

Mark, a cancer patient in his late thirties, resolved, "I want to fight for a longer life, and one with as much quality as possible." He explored treatment options and their side effects, and also asked himself the following questions:

Why do I want to fight?

What is it that I most want to do?

What do I want to experience?

What do I want to complete?

What do I want to heal?

What do I want to resolve?

Mark then chose symbols as reminders of those things that were most important to him: a passport to represent travel, a glass heart for his desire to love again, and an old family photo of a happy time as a symbol for healing a rift within his family. He placed the items on an altar he made in his home. Twice a day Mark reflected on what was most important to him, and this helped him stay focused on why he was fighting for more time. He found this to be especially helpful when treatment fatigue and life's frustrations dragged hard on his spirit. He later added a Swiss army knife as a symbol for cutting through to what was important. His Swiss army knife also served as a reminder that he had an array of "tools" to help him solve whatever problems he encountered.

Interestingly, the word "altar" derives from the Latin word *altus*, meaning high. In a religious setting, it is used as a place for making offerings or consecrating symbols such as wine and bread. Mark used his personal altar as a place to put reminders of things he wanted to keep high in his mind. Altars often hold objects or pictures that lift our spirits and bring them into harmony with a higher good. An altar can be purely psychological, purely spiritual, or a blend of the two.

Mark's altar included spiritual symbols as reminders of his source for guidance, and for soul strength. Yours might include religious symbols, a photo of a public or private person who inspires you, or a scene that evokes peace and inner strength. An altar can serve as a place that physically holds representations of things that you want to be holding in your mind and heart as you move through the ups and downs of life. Your altar should be your own personal creation—made from your highest intentions and hopes.

Letting Go in Grace

Despite the amazing medical advances of recent years, there are circumstances where no treatments are promising enough to be worth the side effects. Such was the case for both my father and my uncle, so they chose not to enter into the medical battle with the disease. It was painful for all of us to accept this fact, but denying it would have been even more painful.

Businessman and author, Eugene O'Kelly, was diagnosed at the age of 53 with an inoperable, malignant brain tumor. In his book, *Chasing Daylight: How My Forthcoming Death Transformed My Life,* he chronicled his diagnosis and what he chose to do with his precious time rather than pursue futile treatment. O'Kelly's memoir opens with these words:

> I was blessed. I was told I had three months to live. [...] I was forced to think seriously about my own death. Which meant I was forced to think more deeply about my life than I'd ever done. Unpleasant as it was, I forced myself to acknowledge that I was in the final stage of life, forced myself to decide how to spend my last 100 days (give or take a few weeks), forced myself to act on those decisions.
>
> In short, I asked myself to answer two questions: Must the end of life be the worst part? And, Can it be made a constructive experience—even the best part of life?

Gene's approach to his death is admirable, and though it was very right for him, it would not be right for everyone. There are aspects of it, though, that you may want to apply to your own decision making process. The great lesson is his ability to look at his own death and not avert his eyes, to openly look at his options and choose what would work best for him.

In many cases, though, one fights for as long, and sometimes longer, than it makes sense to fight. The realization that it is time to let go of the fight may come suddenly, or may be a gradual process.

It is often a rocky transition with great tension between two sides of the self. One side thinks, "I know that I'm going to die before long," and another side says, "I want to push that away and not believe it yet." Tension results from trying to block out truths that nonetheless force themselves upon us. Sometimes we need to believe for just a while longer that recovery is possible. We don't want to let go of hope yet, we want for things to go on the way that they had been. It can be a difficult transition that creates a lot of extra stress, with both patient and caregiver needing to reorient themselves, yet again. We don't want to let go of hope, because then what will we have to hold onto?

Letting go does not have to be a time of abandoning all hope, but it is a time of exchanging one set of hopes for another. Throughout our lives, we trade one hope for something else as circumstances change. A young boy may hope to be a famous ball-player, but as an adult he hopes to get tickets to the World Series. The man who realizes his hope of becoming a pro ballplayer, before long, starts hoping for a better contract and a major endorsement deal.

If you realize you are not going to get better, you don't give up all hope, but what you hope for does change. Ilene said that when she was initially diagnosed with kidney disease, she hoped for a cure and fought hard. When hope for a cure no longer seemed likely, she was initially devastated, but after a while she turned her focus toward hope for a certain quality of life in the time she had left. As her disease progressed, she hoped to live until her grandchild was born. Growing more ill, she told me her hopes were to be free of pain and surrounded with loving care. As she drew closer to the time of her dying, she told me she hoped her life had held meaning for others, and she hoped she would be able to die peacefully at home. Ilene taught me that we keep adjusting our hopes in the dying process, just as we do throughout the rest of our lives.

Another patient who was dying, Elena, had a difficult time accepting that she could no longer plan for next year, or even six months down the road. After resisting this for a while, one afternoon Elena told me that she had realized that resisting the truth of her situation was causing her more pain than accepting it would cause her. She resolved to come to terms with her impending death: "I can't plan for next year, but I can plan for my last days. And that's my next project."

Elena knew that I was writing a book, and we occasionally talked about it. Together, we came up with questions that she thought would be helpful for others nearing the end of their lives.

What is left undone in practical terms, as well as in relationships?

What is left unfulfilled in me that perhaps could be fulfilled? Even if this could only happen in a partial way, what would help me to feel a greater sense of wholeness?

Is there anything I need to resolve before leaving this earth?

In the time left me, while I can still actively participate in life, what do I most need and want to do?

What do I hope my last days will be like?

Where do I want to be?

Are there special aspects of my surroundings that would be important?

Who do I want to be with me?

Is there particular music I think I'd want to be listening to?

Are there prayers I would want said?

What guided meditations or visualizations do I think would be helpful?

What do I hope for between now and then?

What is left to do that must be taken care of so that I can be at peace with my life?

If you are not already involved with a palliative care team, you would do well to request that support. As mentioned previously, a palliative care team can help alleviate many symptoms and assist with pain control if needed. Hospice is also an incredible resource to help patients and caregivers live better as they move through what is often a difficult, yet potentially a richly rewarding time.

Transition Ritual

There are times when family members can't accept that medical treatment will not be sufficiently effective to warrant the side effects, and so they urge patients to keep fighting. Just as the patient's decision on the course of treatment should be respected, each patient has the right to choose to discontinue treatment. Each patient needs to honor their own body, and their own values. There are circumstances when it makes sense to let go of the fight and accept that the body is too ill. It is okay to let go of the struggle for "more" and focus instead on doing what there is in this "now" with graceful acceptance.

One way to be graceful is to practice gratitude. Sit quietly and allow gratitude for the past to fill your heart. Also, practice gratitude for the present, and for the future. At first glance, one might think, *Grateful? How could I be grateful?* But there are many ways to focus on the healing power of gratitude.

Anne's early treatment sent her cancer into remission. Several years later it returned and treatment was not successful. Anne discovered that focusing on gratitude smoothed her transition into acceptance of her situation. She created an altar of thanks and placed symbols of all she had done that was important to her following her initial diagnosis: a photo of herself at the top of a mountain she had climbed, the birth announcement of her first grandchild, a small vase of flowers from the garden she'd planted. In the center of her altar she put a few symbols of what she hoped for in the time left her: a small book in which she was recording her favorite memories of her family, an icon that represented her faith, a figurine of a family hugging one another, and a silly wind-up frog to symbolize laughter.

One man whose eyesight was failing had times of despair over this loss, but at the same time he was still grateful that for most of his life he'd had good vision. He had seen so much; the Taj Mahal bathed in moonlight, sunlight dancing on his granddaughter's copper hair, bright yellow daffodils nodding in the breeze. He was deeply appreciative that these images and so many more were still vivid in his memories. And he was grateful that even though he could only dimly make out the shape of his wife, still, he could clearly hear her voice and be soothed by her touch.

While on an international flight, Joan panicked when there was engine trouble and she feared the plane might go down. *There are so many things left undone,* she thought. When the plane landed safely, she intended to do all of those things, but after taking care of only a few, she got distracted by the demands of everyday life. When Joan was diagnosed with cancer ten years later she felt that she was given another chance to address some important issues before she died. As each one was completed, she offered thanks at having had the opportunity to do so.

Margaret discovered her situation provided her with gratitude. She was most grateful that her family deeply cared about her, and she them. A more surprising source of gratitude was realizing her dying would not involve leaving the person she loved most—her husband, who had died several years earlier. In fact, she was grateful that she would have the pull toward her husband to help her across the great divide. And while she felt great sadness at leaving this earth, her death held the promise of reunion with her beloved husband and she was most thankful for the comfort this offered.

While some individuals feel a lessening of stress through facing their death, there are others who approach their dying by denying it because that is less stressful for them. That is their choice, and their choices are to be respected. All of us, though, can focus on gratitude for the living moment.

CHAPTER 6

Gathering with Friends and Family

Calling together family and friends can be healing. Invite them to be a part of your journey forward, no matter whether it is likely to take you toward recovery or toward the end of life. The gathering can be small or large. The important thing is to surround yourself with love and support.

There are those who have thrown a big party shortly after their diagnosis. One went so far as to call it a "still-living wake." Knowing that friends and family would some day come together at the funeral, one patient stated she wanted to gather with those she cared about while still able to enjoy their company. A party like this would be perfect for some people. If you're one of them, go for it. Make it extravagant, modest, or charity focused, whatever you want it to be.

A party didn't feel quite right to Mary, a woman in her sixties, but she wanted to do something. She accepted that there was little that could be done to battle her cancer and she didn't want those around her pretending she would be okay. Together, we came up with this invitation:

*You are invited to a gathering of close
friends and family*

*to honor the truth that my life is
coming to an end.*

*There are many things for which I want to
say, "Thank you,"*

*and a few things for which
I want to say, "I'm sorry."*

*I also want to share a few favorite stories
with you,*

*and I hope that in turn you
will share with me.*

In notes at the bottom of the invitations, Mary requested that each person bring a special dish that she particularly liked. In part, because Mary wanted to taste her favorite foods again while she still had an appetite. She also wanted to give her friends and family something to do for her, which she knew would help make them feel better.

Mary thought it would be less awkward if people knew ahead of time what to expect, and the invitation gave people time to think about things they wanted to say and stories they'd like to share. By addressing her impending death, Mary cued people as to how she wanted to deal with it. By offering some guidance, Mary helped her friends and family to feel more comfortable with her.

While this could certainly be done more casually, Mary had soft lighting in her living room and a candle for each person present.

She took the lead and started by lighting her candle, symbolically sharing her light as she verbalized her gratitude. As each person had a turn, he or she lit a candle, shared the light, and offered gratitude. By the time they had gone around the circle, there was a sense of warm openness and intimacy. This paved the way and made it easier to move into harder stuff. As they went around the circle again, they shared regrets and apologies. Most were about small things, but there were a few bigger things, too.

And then came the stories, wonderful stories. Some evoked awe, others laughter, some brought a few tears, but the stories made the sharing of the food even more of a communion among them as they moved into eating halfway through the storytelling.

However you might choose to adapt this ritual, it works best if this same order is followed. "Thank you" is easy to say, and sharing gratitude is heartwarming for everyone. "I'm sorry" or "I'm sad" is harder, sometimes involving deeper feelings that might not be able to find expression otherwise. The sharing of stories then lifts people back into more upbeat interactions. The ritual provides a way into, and then a way up out of the "deep stuff."

Usually, it's okay to go into issues with some tension around them, if it's done with the intent and true spirit of resolving it rather than venting anger or resentment. In most situations, such an exchange can be greatly healing for everyone. There was a particularly thorny issue with one of Mary's sisters that she decided not to address in front of the others. It was easier, though, for both women to talk about it on a later occasion because of the gathering a week earlier— they had practiced healing the hurts that can accompany conflicting points of view.

Of course, a similar sharing could be done on an individual basis, but it might be easier to open the door for everyone at the same time with a gathering for this purpose. And once the door is opened, people may feel more comfortable being honest with the situation, and one another, in the time that follows.

David, a man in his mid-thirties who had a good shot at beating his cancer, wanted a different kind of gathering. His invitation read:

My diagnosis caused so many things in life to shift.

What has held true are the connections with family and friends.

Your love and support over the past two months has touched me deeply, and has fueled my desire to fight this disease.

You are invited to a gathering to help nourish me for the journey ahead.

I would love you to bring _____ for a pot-luck dinner.

I would also like you to bring two stories to share:

1. Something you've learned from me.

2. A funny story of something that happened when we were together.

He preferred to skip the candles and the deeper level of addressing regrets, wanting to keep the evening more upbeat, which was how he wanted to deal with his illness. Like Mary, cueing others as to how he felt about his diagnosis allowed his friends and family to feel more comfortable around him.

Alison didn't want a gathering, but she did want to reach out and connect with special people in her life. She wrote a dozen or so letters that began:

> *My diagnosis made me see how precarious is life. This was frightening to me, overwhelming at times. But my illness has also brought me to see how precious are the connections of heart, and of blood, but especially those with whom I feel soul connection. I sometimes become overwhelmed with the value of those I hold dearest. I wish I could tell you this face to face, but since I am so easily overwhelmed these days, I'm afraid I'd never be able to get through it. I do, though, want to tell you how much you, and our relationship, means to me.*

She followed this with a page or more to each person. Most of the recipients wrote Alison in response and told her how important she had been in their lives. Alison loved being able to pull out their letters and re-read them when she felt overwhelmed by all that she was going through.

Kay didn't think she wanted to do anything along these lines. But not long after hearing about the ritual, her friend Susan drove her to the clinic for a chemo treatment. As the IV dripped, Kay told Susan how much she appreciated Susan graciously helping her through aspects of the treatment. Suddenly she remembered a time when Susan had encouraged her to try something new and it had opened up her life in unexpected ways. "I would never have done that if it weren't for you."

Susan was pleased to know that this had meant so much to Kay, and it prompted Susan to relate something important that Kay had done for her.

As they sat there smiling at one another in grateful understanding, Kay remembered the sequence of the ritual and realized that she wanted to apologize to Susan for something she'd done that had bothered her off and on for years. This seemed an appropriate opportunity, so she took a deep breath, revealed her transgression, and asked forgiveness. Susan not only forgave her, but reciprocated with her own confession and apology. The women cried and hugged, then they laughed and hugged. They easily slid into a lovely time of "Remember when …," which not only kept them both entertained for the rest of the chemo treatment session, but brought them closer than they'd felt since Kay's diagnosis.

CHAPTER 7

Outlets for Anger and Grief

While we may sometimes be philosophical about our circumstances, other times we're filled with rage. Sometimes the anger is small and specific: frustration with a mistake at the pharmacy, or irritation with someone's ignorant and insensitive remark. Sometimes, the anger is larger and amorphous: rage at God or our body for failing us. Sometimes, it is the complicated anger we feel toward a loved one. Other times, we don't know why we are angry—we just are! In all of these cases, we need a safe way to express the anger so we can get to what is underneath the difficult feelings.

Sometimes after venting the anger we can then let it go. If not, maybe there is something that can be done. For instance, my irritation with the pharmacy and its mistakes prompted me to always check the bottles before I left the store. Sometimes there is a lesson to be learned, or insight to be recognized, in situations that initially make us angry. Other times, it's just one of those frustrating things in life we have to deal with.

When Anger Surfaces

The first step when anger wells up in you is to find a constructive way to let it out. Often, it helps to have a ritual that creates a safe space for the expression of these feelings.

One way to do so is to affirm that part of being alive means having a wide range of thoughts and feelings. We all experience fear, anger, and sorrow throughout our lives in response to a variety of situations. These are natural responses and part of being human. If we give expression to these feelings, then we don't have to carry so much of it around inside us.

Sometimes anger flies out of us, and other times it can be difficult to express. You may find it helpful to say out loud, "Part of being alive means being angry sometimes, and right now I'm angry. I am so angry because ...." Then allow yourself to vent the anger in a way that is comfortable for you, and not hurtful to anyone else. Shout it to the bathroom walls, hit a pillow, tell someone who will simply listen to how angry you are. There are many ways to express anger.

Barbara and her husband bought a hand drum and as they pounded on it they chanted and shouted their anger, letting the thoughts and feelings rise up and out of them through their mouths and their hands. In the process, they discovered they had rage about many things they hadn't realized. Simply being aware of it helped. They also discovered that beneath their anger was love—love for one another, and love for the life they shared. Periodically releasing their anger allowed them to clear some of it away so they could connect more strongly to the love. Sometimes their anger gave way to grief. Sharing the grief helped each of them individually, and brought them even closer as a couple.

Banging on a drum doesn't work for everyone, though there can be something wonderfully therapeutic in it, and a drum often works better than hitting a pillow. The drum's sounds fill out the words we say, especially when we can't find the right words. Move into the anger by repeating, "I hate this, I hate this, I hate this ...." And then list your angers. If your mind goes blank, you can simply go back to repeating, "I hate this, I hate this." Go back to chanting it anytime you don't have words to express the specifics. It can help you move into a place of honesty. You may feel self-conscious for the first minute or so, but gradually you will connect to something deeper than thought, and this allows for genuine release, and often a clearer insight into your anger.

Some might prefer to write down their anger, others paint or draw it, while still others will express themselves through music. Experiment with different methods. Even if you haven't painted since kindergarten, you can simply allow the feelings to come through in whatever colors and shapes flow out on the paper or canvas. Experimenting in an area where you're a total novice can be therapeutic, and often more enlightening than an area where you have a certain expertise, in part because you'll be less inclined to feel a need to do it well.

Pam, an artist in her forties, resisted writing her thoughts until one day she put down her paintbrush and picked up a pen. I had encouraged her to try an exercise of "free writing," a method where grammar, punctuation, and spelling are of no importance; all that matters is to keep the hand moving. The purpose is to not consciously think what word is going to come next, but to allow uncensored thoughts and feelings to flow forth unhampered. Pam found the results of this kind of writing to be more interesting than she'd expected. One afternoon she wrote:

> *There are times when I am angry at everyone who is still healthy, angry that they can concern themselves with finding the right pair of shoes. Sometimes I'm angry with those who are trying to take care of me because—I don't know why, but sometimes I am. There are times that I hate*

my body for betraying me. Times I curse the fates for bringing
this to me now. I am angry that I didn't do certain things
before this. I'm angry with my family for visiting but not
participating. And I'm angry with me for not being able to
handle it the way I want to be handling it.

Her last line held the most energy for her, and Pam felt that
perhaps that was underneath much of her other anger. We talked
about how she thought she should be handling it. Then, together
we assessed how realistic her expectations were. Pam discovered
she needed to be more compassionate with herself, so she shifted
her expectations to be less demanding and more in alignment with
who she was. Sometimes we soar, sometimes we stumble. We're
human.

Once you get the anger out, look at it, and perceive any grief
that might be underneath. Listen to your anger and grief—at the very
least, the feelings want to be acknowledged. You may discover there
are certain things you can do to have some control over the future,
however radically altered it may be from what you wanted. Similar to
the story about John writing letters to his children in Chapter 3, the
anger can be a gift that helps you see what could be done.

Just as we need a way into anger, we also need a way to move out
of it. One way to close an anger ritual is to take several long, slow,
deep breaths, and allow yourself to let go of the angry feelings—at
least for now.

Breathe in through your nose, give a big exhale through your
mouth, and visualize the anger leaving your body.

Repeat this slow steady breathing several times until you've let
go of all that you can for right now. Then say aloud, "Even though
I have anger, I'm still so grateful for ...," and focus on something

that inspires real gratitude. Take a few moments to rest and breathe in gratitude.

There is something truly remarkable about connecting with our gratitude. It isn't an antidote for anger or pain, but it reminds us that despite the difficulties, there is much in life that supports us, and brings us joy. Focusing on the positive aspects of our lives can help bring us into balance. When our path takes us through difficult terrain, we need to do all we can to keep our balance.

The Forgiving Pot

Just the idea of an anger ritual gives us permission to be angry. It sanctions the feelings. If none of the previous suggestions work for you, you may discover the perfect approach to dealing with your anger on your own. Just open yourself to the possibility.

Cynthia, a woman whose husband was dying, asked me for an anger ritual. We discussed a number of ideas, but none of them felt quite right to her. I suggested she just keep it all in mind, and see what occurred to her. Several days later a friend gave her a decorative pot. Cynthia decided the pot could be a receptacle for her anger and frustration. She could write down her anger and then put the paper inside the pot. If she said she hated God or her husband, the pot would know that she didn't really mean it, she was just angry. She called it her Forgiving Pot.

A week or so later when I asked her about it, she said she hadn't written anything, but when she was angry the pot became a place to focus that energy. She shouted at the pot, she gave it mean looks, sometimes her hatred of certain things would be aimed across the room and into the pot. Wonderfully, the pot was not only a receptacle for her anger, it also offered forgiveness for the anger. One day, Cynthia told me, "This pot makes it so much easier for me to express my anger whenever it comes up, and then let it go."

Often, underneath our anger is grief. There are a number of losses that may cause grief: loss of normalcy, loss of innocence, loss of illusions, loss of independence, loss of the future we wanted for ourselves and others. As with anger, it is helpful to allow ourselves space to grieve. Talk it through, cry, write it, paint it, sing it, sit with it.

After the grief has been honored, let it flow out of you. Breathe deeply and let it go. Then breathe in gratitude. Focus on gratitude for a new sense of priorities; gratitude that people show how much they care, gratitude for a new openness. And if there is something you can do about the grief, as John did in writing letters to his children, be grateful that you have found an avenue for meaningful expression.

CHAPTER 8

Taking Care of One's Self

So much time and energy is spent attending to medical needs that we think we're very focused on taking care of ourselves. But there is more to the self than just the body, and there is more to taking care of the body than just addressing the disease. The whole self wants and needs attention, and this holds true not only for patients, but also for family members—especially the primary caregiver whose needs are often pushed to the side. Keeping a sense of balance in life requires that we take time to relax, experience pleasure, connect with a larger world—and our larger self.

Take a Break

A favorite ritual to relax and reconnect is simple and easy. Take a break. *Really* take a break. Leave the house and go for a walk. Don't take anything with you, except a special friend, perhaps. Leave the cell phone behind, along with your worries. The key moment is when you shut the door. Firmly close it as a symbolic gesture that you are leaving everything inside the house, bringing nothing of it with you when you go out.

One gentleman told me he could feel all the "stuff" in his life wanting to come with him when he took a walk, just like a puppy not wanting to be left behind. He would say aloud as he was backing out the door, "You can't come with me right now. You stay here. Stay!" If any of the distracting thoughts tried to follow him, he'd send them back home like a bad dog, sternly ordering, "Go home! Go on, go!"

I have had people ask, "If I don't think about any of what I usually think about, what do I think about?"

Don't think, just notice the world around you. Allow yourself to simply be in the moment. Even circling the block, or just up to the corner and back, pay attention to things you usually don't notice. How does the sun feel on your skin? Listen closely to the many different sounds. Become aware of the odd symphony that is created by cars, the wind, voices, barking dogs—all the sounds that come in and fall away like instruments in an orchestra. Pay attention to details. Notice flowers, the larger landscape, interesting architecture. Look for what is different from last week, or what you've never noticed before. What's always the same? One day pay particular attention to subtle smells, the next focus on something else.

Being mindful of the world outside of you helps you take a total break from all that normally preoccupies you. Mindfulness also invites you to open yourself to the world in a different way. In the process, you might start to open yourself to your Self in a different way, too.

This kind of mindful break provides psychological and physical benefits. In the 1800s, it was customary to take a morning or evening "constitutional," a stroll through the neighborhood to breathe fresh air and get a bit of exercise. When time and energy are limited, as they often are during medical treatments, a walk around the block might be the only way to work in a bit of gentle exercise. While not a serious workout, the health benefits are measurable. It helps maintain muscle strength, and the relaxed, rhythmic movement calms the body and psyche.

Focusing your attention on immediate surroundings is a little bit like mindfulness meditation, so, sometimes be aware of your breath, how it feels as you inhale and exhale. Notice how the pavement or earth feels beneath your feet, or how the muscles in your legs feel as they stretch and contract.

Even after walking became difficult for my husband, thanks to a wheelchair, we could still take our evening constitutional. Tony missed the exercise, but appreciated the fresh air and change of scenery as I wheeled him around the neighborhood. Many of the people I've worked with have found this ritual to be pleasant, helpful, and well worth the small investment of time and energy. Give it a try.

Setting Boundaries

When Tony began to need more rest, we carved space into his afternoons for a nap. In addition, we avoided planning anything for several days following his treatments so he could rest and recover. There were regular doctors' appointments, radiation or chemo treatments, and weekly blood draws. Tony liked to have time in the morning to ease into the day, so whenever possible, we avoided scheduling any appointments in the early morning. We were simply doing what seemed practical. I realize now we were also setting boundaries to honor what was necessary and important as well as honoring Tony's personal needs and rhythms.

As we made schedule adjustments to accommodate all of the additional demands on our time, Tony suggested that we keep Sundays completely open and have it truly be a day off from everything. But Sunday was the day that was most convenient for his family to visit, and I wanted him to feel their love and support, so that took up a big chunk of the day. On the rare occasions when his family didn't visit, we took advantage of the opening to see a friend who was only able to visit on Sundays.

I wanted Tony to feel as much support as possible from all directions—that was a priority. Yet, I now wish we had periodically said "no" to everyone and really taken the full day off just to kick back and simply move through the day as the spirit moved us. It would have served both of us very well to have such a respite at least once a month. We certainly could have done so. It would not have been terrible for us to take one Sunday a month to ourselves, and one other weekend a month asked his family to come on Saturday so we could see our friend on that Sunday. In hindsight, I now see we could have catered to others a little less and catered to ourselves a little more.

If there are areas of your life where this is occurring, it is important to take a step back, realize that it's impossible to do everything, and then see what is most important to you right now.

In Marjorie Williams's book, *Woman at the Washington Zoo*, she writes about the time following her diagnosis with liver cancer. She describes a phone conversation with a good friend, and as they excitedly planned to get together for lunch, Marjorie looked at her calendar and realized:

> *...there will only be about seven [free] hours before the next treatment. I am forced to admit that in this cramped context, I don't actually want to spend two of those hours with the person I'm talking to. These forced choices make one of the biggest losses of sickness.*
>
> *But on the other side of this coin is a gift. I think cancer brings to most people a new freedom to act on the understanding that their time is important. My editor at The Washington Post told me, when I first got sick, that after his mother recovered from cancer his parents literally never went anywhere they didn't want to. If you have ever told yourself, breezily, that life is too short to spend any of it with your childhood neighbor's annoying husband, those words now take on the gleeful raiment of simple fact. The*

knowledge that time's expenditure is important, that it is
up to you, is one of the headiest freedoms you will ever feel.

Time is precious, and it makes sense to use it well. To do so, you need to be honest with yourself about what your true priorities are at this point in your life. Perhaps one of the great gifts of facing a serious illness is the opportunity to cut through the "shoulds" and identify what really matters. To help you find your priorities, write down your responses to the following:

Experiences in my life that
    are necessary
    nourish me
    teach me
    inspire me
    soothe me
    refresh me
    bring me deep pleasure
    fill me with love and gratitude

Experiences in my life that
    feel obligatory
    drain me
    seem like an utter waste of time

Resolve to say "no" to as many items as possible on the second list so you can say "yes" to more things that enrich and enliven you. The following ritual can help you to connect with that resolve. Have someone slowly read it while you focus on the images and sensations. (An audio of this visualization is also available on my website at: www.healingthroughillness.com.)

Sitting in a chair, plant your feet on the ground. Close your eyes and imagine roots spreading out from the soles of your feet and reaching down into the earth. They are reaching down so that they can draw up into yourself the nourishment that you need. Say "yes" to this nourishment with everything within you.

Feel that nourishment flowing into you through your feet and spreading up through your legs. Let this life-giving sap move up and spread out through your torso. Feel it coming up into your head, and flowing out through your arms all the way down to your fingertips.

Experience that vital sap strengthening and sweetening your fullest being.

Feel it flowing through your body, its life-giving properties coursing through your veins. Allow yourself to bask in this for as long as you like.

This is what saying "yes" to your first list does for you, on more levels than you may realize. Give yourself permission to say "no" to the things that prevent you from saying "yes" to as many of the first list items as possible.

Envision yourself erecting boundaries around those things that you most want to protect, and as you do so, think about why. Allow yourself to fully understand that it is important to preserve time for those things that strengthen and sweeten vitality.

Open your eyes and make space and time right now for at least half an hour of doing something that nourishes you.

A Special Note to Caregivers

It is essential that caregivers set boundaries, too. While it is legitimate for the patient's needs to take precedence most of the time, it is essential that this doesn't happen *all* of the time. When someone you love is very ill, his care becomes more important than anything else. My job, taking care of the house, cooking, laundry, and running errands, were scheduled around Tony's needs as much as possible. Only if there was a bit of open space did I even think of my own needs.

In retrospect, I can see it would have been good for me to establish some boundaries to take care of myself as well. It seems appropriate that 80 percent of the focus was on Tony, but when less than 5 percent of the focus was on me and my needs, things were too far out of balance.

For many years, I had practiced yoga for thirty minutes, four or five times a week, but after Tony got sick I only managed to do yoga four or five times a year. After not feeding my inner self for so long, one day when I reached for a creative solution for Tony's needs, I came up empty. The well inside was dry. I realized that for Tony's sake I needed to feed me. After that, I attended a writing workshop for four months, one evening a week, and that provided me with what I needed. Probably, it would have been good for me to have continued with the class longer, but I hated imposing on others to stay with Tony for more Monday nights than was absolutely necessary.

Almost a year after Tony's diagnosis, I had two people say the same thing to me within the same week: "Every time I ask how you are, you tell me how Tony is doing. I want to know how you are."

I responded, "How Tony is doing, is how I am."

Not long after that, though, I started seeing a therapist. I felt I needed someone to help keep me in balance so I could help Tony keep his balance as we moved through the difficulties. For one hour a week therapy forced me to focus on myself, pay attention to my thoughts and feelings, and address some of my own needs. My therapist helped me to keep some sense of a context that went beyond Tony's care. And taking care of myself helped me to take better care of Tony.

Often, I had reminded young, overworked mothers that on an airplane the flight attendants always instruct passengers, "In case of an emergency, put on your own oxygen mask first."

I told these moms, "If you don't take care of you, how are you going to take care of anyone else?"

Wise words that I somehow forgot in the thick of caring for Tony. At one point, some of those same women reminded me of this sage advice. I understood it intellectually, but because Tony's life was at stake, I wanted to focus on him. Though there were many days I didn't have time for even a quick shower, and never ever got enough sleep, it was hard for me to realize that I was ignoring some of my most basic needs. I encourage you to make time for what is necessary for your optimal functioning. Even when the care of another is the most important priority, don't fall into the habit of foregoing your own basic needs.

Because I know so well the difficulties involved, I developed ways for caregivers to seamlessly slip some self-care into their daily schedules. The following chapter offers suggestions on finding time to relax for both patient and caregiver.

CHAPTER 9

Relaxation Rituals

Serious illness is stressful for patients and their caregivers, so it is important to take special time to relax. Meditation CDs or visualizations that guide us into a place of deep relaxation can provide an interlude of tranquility to help maintain strength and sanity.

I know it is hard to find the time, but if patient and caregiver make a ritual of relaxing together, it is more likely to happen. Set aside a specific time for this every day if you can, but at least once a week. Take time afterward to talk quietly together without feeling rushed to jump back into all the things that need to be done. It can be a special time of intimacy and easy conversation.

Taking little relaxation breaks throughout the day is also important, especially on the days when there isn't time for a relaxation break. No matter how demanding our schedule is, we can find time for several mini-breaks every day to relax. The space for these breaks is there in our daily routine just waiting for us to take advantage of the moments.

For instance, washing our hands is one of the best ways to protect ourselves and others from infection. To thoroughly wash our hands, we are encouraged to scrub them for forty-five seconds—as long as it takes to sing "Happy Birthday" twice. Taking half a dozen long, slow breaths while washing your hands doesn't take any longer, yet can provide you with an oasis of calm. If you consciously release muscle tension and let go of frustrations when you exhale, you can use the time to help relieve stress.

The following meditation will help you turn hand washing into a much needed a relaxation break. Post a copy of the Bathroom Meditation near your bathroom sink to help remind you to thoroughly wash your hands at least twice a day, and totally relax for 45 seconds.

Bathroom Meditation

As you put your hands under the running water, let go of tension from your face down to your feet.

While soaping your hands take a slow, deep breath and as you exhale, consciously let go of more tension. Allow it to sink down and out through the soles of your feet.

Let all remaining stress and worry flow down into your hands.

Now massage your hands, first the palms, then move the tension out to your fingertips, massaging each finger as you gently scrub. Allow for at least three long, slow, deep breaths as you do this.

As you rinse your hands, let the tension wash down the drain.

Reach for the towel, and take another long, deep breath to further restore you to yourself. And then one more breath to give you clarity and energy to better deal with what's in front of you.

A particularly good time to do the Bathroom Meditation is when you first come home after having been out in the world—

usually having picked up both germs and tension. No matter how full your day is you really can afford to spend a whole minute to breathe in serenity and wash away the germs and tension.

At other times, utilize even the quickest hand washing to remind you to at least take a few long, slow, deep breaths and let go of tension in your body. Before long, washing your hands becomes a tiny, but regular space to consciously relax your body and relieve some of life's stress.

While none of the relaxation rituals will totally eliminate tension, they will lessen it, and if you do them often enough, you can keep stress from taking too great a toll.

Bedtime Meditation

At the end of the day when you crawl into bed, a good way to relax and let go of the day's worries is a simple meditation ritual. To easily learn this little ritual, take the first line only for a few nights, and take half a dozen slow breaths to explore the full feeling of it. Then add another line, exploring the feelings evoked by that phrase or image for three or four nights.

Continue adding phrases until you are familiar with all of the lines. And of course, alter the wording in whatever way feels appropriate to better address your needs. I find it helpful to consciously tense and relax my entire body two or three times before beginning the meditation. At night before falling asleep, slowly say any or all of the following lines with one long, slow breath in between.

For this space of time, I can let go of all the stress.
   I let go of tension from my face down to my feet.
   I can let go of all that weighs me down.
   I can let go of all that drains me.
   I let go, I let go, I let go.
From now until morning, all I need to do is breathe.
This breathing nourishes me
   from the soles of my feet,
   to the crown of my head,
   to the center of my being.

Anytime Meditation

I have found this meditation helpful to find a place of calm centeredness, whether I am in a waiting room, stopped at a red light, pacing hospital corridors, or waiting for water to boil.

I open myself and allow God's light to flow into me.
Opening myself fully, I allow God's love to shine
   through me.

(If "God's light" isn't a phrase that is right for you, replace it with whatever is: white light, the mother light of Buddha consciousness, or the light in your loved one's eyes.)

This meditation can be done for ten seconds, two minutes, or an hour. Just keep breathing in the light and the love, let them flood into each cell in your body, filling you heart, mind, and soul. Then let the light and love flow out from you into the world. Sometimes, I say the first line three times, then the second line three times, and do three sets of this. Play with it to see what works best for you.

Regularly give yourself the gift of time and space to relax and restore your body, mind, heart and spirit—even if it's only a few minutes twice a day. In an ideal world, we would have thirty to forty minutes every day for deep relaxation, plus several five-minute breaks. But even the minimum of one longer session a week and two short relaxation breaks a day can make a big difference. During great difficulty in life, we need to offer ourselves compassion and nurturing so we can move through life's challenges with as much strength and grace as possible.

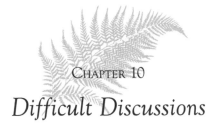

CHAPTER 10

Difficult Discussions

$\mathcal{M}$any people feel it is important to discuss their thoughts about the process of dying and their beliefs relating to death. Talking about the larger context of life often brings meaning into the journey. But some people may be unsure how to bring up the subject, or even if they should.

Often, people find themselves veering away from it. There are so many questions and fears: What if talking about death is painful or depressing? How will the other person react? How will I react if I really get into talking about it? What if we cry?

These are understandable concerns. You may cry; the thought of leaving, or being left, is sad. But if you can discuss your worries and fears, they will weigh less heavily on your mind and heart. In many cases, sharing the pain can help both patient and caregiver to bear it all a little better.

Yet, even those who have talked at length about death and dying prior to diagnosis find it is suddenly different when death is no longer hypothetical. Oftentimes, people have an irrational fear that talking about death might make it happen. But saying the words out loud won't make it happen anymore than not addressing death can prevent it from happening.

Some years after my dad died, my mom told me, "We talked about death periodically before he got sick, sometimes in terms of spirituality, and sometimes as an inevitability for us both. But we didn't talk about it really after his diagnosis. I wanted to talk about it, but I didn't know if I should bring it up—I thought it might upset him. He probably wanted to talk about it, too, and thought the same thing about not wanting to upset me. I wish we had talked about his death after he got sick. I think it would have helped both of us."

In this heart-to-heart conversation, my mom admitted, "I guess we were both a little silly to be afraid of bringing it up, afraid to upset the other person—as if either of us might have forgotten all about it! As if his impending death wasn't uppermost on both of our minds!"

For various reasons we sidestep talking about death. In my case, I wanted my husband to stay positive, believing a positive attitude could help in the miracle of healing. Instead, what I did was leave him alone with his fears. While we did talk about the possibility of his death on occasion, I was usually too intent on pulling Tony back to a more optimistic frame of mind. Now, I understand Tony needed me to sit with him and keep him company as he explored his thoughts and feelings about what he was facing, and what he might face in the future.

Tony didn't need me to "fix" it, and he didn't need me to banish his thoughts and fears about dying. I think he wanted me to explore the subject with him as we had explored so much else in our discussions over the years. Now, I wish we had had those conversations; sharing our thoughts and feelings would have been an interesting and meaningful experience for both of us.

I have thought a lot about why I wasn't willing to fully enter into those discussions and I have wondered: Was it only wanting to keep our eyes focused on the bull's eye of survival with the single-mindedness of a Zen archer? Was some of my reluctance because I was afraid he would have questions for which I had no answers?

Was I afraid that if I looked at his dying squarely in the face, I might collapse and my resolve to move forward through it would dissolve? Or was I afraid I would melt into such a mass of tears that Tony would feel overwhelmed wanting to fix my sorrow, and at the same time a little bit angry or resentful that I was falling apart when he needed me to be there for him? I was probably afraid of all of these things and more.

I wouldn't have had answers to all of his questions, though I could answer some of them a little better now. (Later in this chapter I offer some of those answers.) What we both missed in not going there together was the chance to share in the uncertainty and fear and anguish together. Each of us could have been there for the other, sharing the grief, sometimes crying together, holding one another. Might it have sometimes been just awful? Possibly, but even at its worst, probably not worse than pushing the thought of death away when it needed to be addressed more fully. These intimate conversations would likely have nourished both of us, and brought us even closer.

Impending death has its own particular light, and it casts a different kind of illumination upon the world. It makes sense to talk about how different so many things look when you or someone you love is making this passage. Your attitudes and feelings may well be altered, or even radically changed in certain respects from what they were a year ago. This makes it even more important to explore what your thoughts and feelings are *now*.

Ritual for Talking About Death

Sometimes it helps to create special space for the patient and the caregiver to openly and honestly talk about their thoughts, feelings, and concerns. Ritual can provide a way into these conversations, and a way out of them. Participating in such a ritual can provide us with connection to our deeper selves, and to the deeper self of another.

One ritual I developed grew out of the realization that not addressing the prospect of dying weighs on us and can make us feel like we are carrying around a heavy stone. One of my clients, Carol, knew there was no hope of a cure for her disease and she grappled with many difficult feelings. I suggested she find a rock to symbolize this heaviness. She found one that weighed a few pounds—heavy enough that she felt its weight, but not so heavy that it was uncomfortable to hold as she talked, meditated, or wrote in her journal. Over time, Carol saw the stone as a reminder that if she went into her depths, she would find her bedrock and discover what supported her with the same strength as the earth.

When feeling the weight of her concerns, Carol picked up the rock and in doing so, externalized her heavy feelings. She said she felt as if she were literally holding the feelings outside of herself, and this allowed her to be a little more objective and see them more clearly. When Carol finished exploring her thoughts about death, she put the rock down—literally and metaphorically letting go of the heaviness she had been carrying around.

One couple used a special rock as a ritual signal to invite deep discussion. For them, it provided a way to move into exploring their fears, the larger context of life, the metaphysical aspects of death, and the meaning in the dying process. Paul would place the rock on the dining room table to signify he needed to talk about the heavy stuff. As soon as his wife was able, she would pick up the rock and take it to him asking, "Is now a good time for you to talk?"

Selecting a rock may help you gain a better understanding of what questions and concerns weigh you down. Deciding how you will use this symbol to communicate with yourself or a partner will help you clarify how you want this process to work for you. When you are ready to talk on a deeper level, pick up the rock and allow yourself the freedom to express what is weighing upon you. Below are suggestions for topics you may want to explore.

Before diagnosis, my fears and worries were:
Now my fears and worries are about:

This is what I used to think about death and dying:
My thoughts and feelings about it now are:

What do I believe is the larger context of my life?
What are the small and large miracles my heart hopes for?

My fears about the last days and hours are:
My wishes about the last days and hours are:

Allow the conversation to go in whatever direction it needs to go. You probably won't want to address all of these questions in one session, so return to this when there is a need. Also, keep in mind that your responses may change and evolve as you move through the process, so it may be helpful to revisit some of these discussions from time to time. When you have finished the conversation, put the rock aside or return it to its place, then spend a few moments expressing gratitude to one another. This rock ritual may also work with extended family who want to talk, but don't know how or where to begin.

Sometimes, patients are more comfortable talking with a friend, therapist, nurse, or minister, and that's fine, especially if those closest aren't willing or able. The same holds true for caregivers. If your loved one isn't ready to engage in deep discussion, but you need to talk, find someone you trust. Each person's rhythm and timing needs to be respected.

Answers to Questions Difficult to Ask

There are questions people often have, and yet, they find it difficult to ask medical providers. I have answered two of the most common questions below. If you have other questions, I hope you will ask an appropriate person. The gnawing concern of not knowing can be far worse over the long term than finding the courage to ask the question, and hear the answer.

What is it like to die?

The deaths I have witnessed—in hospitals, at home, and even an accident site on the highway—have all been peaceful. The illnesses were sometimes painful, but the dying itself appeared to be simple, effortless. I know it can be otherwise, depending on the circumstances, but usually if the person is in a hospital or in hospice, there is little or no pain. There may be a struggle for breath toward the last, but it is more a reaching for it rather than a violent struggle, a wanting to make the effort—even though it is very much an effort. Perhaps there is even a savoring of these last breaths.

We cannot know what will actually be experienced until we reach that moment, but having been present with loved ones and strangers during their last moments has brought me to a place of peace around it. It is not unusual for the person's face to take on a beatific expression at the end. Is it because of experiencing connection with something beyond? Or because of letting go of all the worries of life? Whatever your beliefs, there is something holy in the moment of dying, just as there is in the moment of birth.

What happens physically to the body?

Each of us is different, and illnesses and circumstances vary, but generally, in the last days the various functions of the body weaken. The kidneys, liver, pancreas, and the vast number of things the organs in our bodies do, all slow down. We no longer desire, and can no longer digest food. Eventually, even swallowing a sip of water is more than the body can manage. There may be some discomfort at times, but nurses and other trained personnel can help to alleviate this.

In the slowing down, the body seems to take charge. There isn't strength to will the body to do more than it deems necessary. The mind may be slowing, yet still alert and present. Even if the patient is not fully aware of where he or she is, there is often an awareness of people, sights, and sounds. The senses of smell, touch, and hearing may function more acutely than usual. The body seems to know exactly what it is doing. The body takes care of the dying process, freeing us from the need to know what to do.

Understanding this allows us to focus on what we need and want to do with our time until we reach our final days.

CHAPTER 11

Nurturing One's Spirit

During serious illness there are too many things that cause bad feelings—being stuck with needles, nausea, and profound fatigue, to name only a few. To help counterbalance this, seek out things that cause good feelings, such as gazing at clouds, seeing someone smile in response to your smile, standing in the yard feeling the wind, and listening with all of your senses to the sounds it creates. Find small moments of pleasure, and orchestrate some larger ones. It is important to feed yourself on all levels.

To do any of these things is to make an offering to yourself, and to the person sharing the experience with you. It might be a major event, such as driving into the country for the weekend or attending the ballet. It can also be simple and spontaneous, such as taking thirty minutes on your way home from an appointment to stroll in a garden or sit on a park bench. Or simply step outside to smell the rain.

Nature

Spend time in nature. Take a day to go to a scenic area that is a comfortable drive from where you live. Visit a public garden, or have a picnic at a local park. Even walking along a city block you can find bits of nature—flowers in a window box, weeds struggling up through cracks in the cement, or fruits and vegetables through a shop window. The hunt for evidence of nature in unlikely places can add to the fun. Nature is everywhere, and it is healing to spend time focusing on it, being with it, breathing it in.

Bring nature into your home. Buy some flowers that please your senses, or intrigue you with their shape and color. Ask a friend with a green thumb to create a dish garden or terrarium for you. Design a miniature Japanese garden with sand, rocks, and a tabletop water fountain. Go out in the backyard with a friend or family member and spend five minutes looking up at the night sky.

Connecting to ourselves, and one another, while connecting with nature can feed us in a most soul-satisfying way.

Music and Art

There is something special about hearing live music. It resonates through us in a different way so that our cells hear the music along with our ears. Make plans to attend a concert, opera, or blue grass festival. A worthwhile alternative is sitting quietly in the living room and only listening to music, letting the notes fill every part of the self. Tony and I liked Henryk Gorecki's "Symphony No. 3," because it echoed our sometimes somber, slow state of mind. We also liked Ralph Vaughn Williams' "The Lark Ascending" for its hopefulness. Seek out your favorites, and discover some new pieces.

Watching a dance performance can take us out of ourselves and for a time our own bodies seem stronger and more supple, a little less earthbound.

Spending an afternoon at a museum or gallery can invite us to look at the world through different eyes. We can also learn what our associations are and the ways they influence us. Art can inspire us to trust our own vision of what we see, even if it is different from that of others.

Ask people to send you copies of some of their favorite poems. Not only will you discover a broad range of new pieces, you will likely gain new insight into the individuals who sent them.

Meditation and Prayer

For centuries, these two practices have enhanced the spiritual well being of people all over the world. The positive effects of meditation and prayer on our bodies, along with our mental and emotional well-being, are well documented. A number of studies show that those who pray regularly recover faster from surgery, and report a higher quality of life than patients who do not have some form of faith. Regular meditation lowers blood pressure and boosts immunity. No less important is the benefit of these practices nourishing the soul. Sitting quietly and watching your breath, or listening to your God or higher power, can provide you with a place of peace that feeds and strengthens your spirit.

There are various kinds of meditation, and numerous CDs, that can guide you in a meditation practice. A basic form of meditation is to sit quietly with eyes closed and observe your breath as it moves in and out. That's all there is to it. Sounds simple, and in one sense, it is. However, the mind strays here and there and yonder. That's okay. Just pull your attention back to your breath. Again and again, bring yourself back to your breath. Sit, breathe, and observe the breath. After a while, something happens. Not earth shattering or psychedelic, but rather quiet and simple. In time, you will see meditation's influence is significant. Try it.

Praying is something many have done since childhood, and something some haven't done since then. It, too, is simple. We open our heart and our mind to connect with the divine consciousness that brought this wondrous universe into being. Many traditional prayers begin with offering thanks; gratitude opens the heart. You can begin by giving thanks for what is most precious and beautiful in your life. Then ask for guidance, strength, more time, perfect health, clarity, whatever springs from you. Speak from your heart.

Do not only talk to God—also *listen* to God. Listen with your heart. Be patient, sit in peace, become quiet inside. Listen. Even if you feel you didn't receive what you needed, offer thanks. You may find that an answer comes later in a rather unexpected way.

For those who are not comfortable praying to a higher being, it is still possible, and beneficial, to spend time in a prayerful state. For some, this involves connecting with *your* higher self, for others it is a matter of connecting with a calm self. You might choose to spend five minutes every morning and evening sitting quietly and allowing yourself to be flooded with gratitude and a feeling of fulfillment. You can focus on your intentions, hopes, or wishes, and then move into a state of harmony with your world to increase the odds of bringing those hopes into the flow of your life.

You can practice connecting with loved ones, heart-to-heart, whether they are in the same room or halfway around the world. Let your love for them flow out from your heart, and allow their love to wash over you like liquid sunshine. Allow this to nurture a sense of peace deep within you. Feeling the fullness of love can feed your deepest being, and connect you to a calm strength that allows you to meet life's challenges with greater grace.

Soul Friends

Spending an afternoon with a friend whose company feeds our souls can be worth its weight in gold. There are those people who help us to see ourselves, our lives, and the world more clearly, so that simply being in their presence nurtures us. Two of Tony's casual friendships developed into soul connections, and he found that some other friendships held less for him in his illness. We have to move with the changes.

One of Tony's new soul friends took him to the park once a week and gave him a private yoga lesson tailored to work with his physical limitations. Tony drew great sustenance from these encounters. Going to the symphony with such a person, or hanging out at home having a cup of tea, can bring deep fulfillment that makes the waiting room at the next medical appointment seem less drab even two days later.

Affection

Holding hands, hugging and cuddling rate higher on my list than chocolate. Before Tony's diagnosis, we were private with our displays of affection, but afterward, we hugged and kissed anywhere and in front of anyone, even in checkout lines at the market. Before long, Tony was exchanging hugs with friends from work.

Physical connection with those we care about, quite literally symbolizes our connections of heart, mind, spirit, and history. Embracing or clasping hands is part of greeting and farewell rituals in cultures around the world because it acknowledges and honors the connections that are present on many levels.

This affirming ritual expression of emotional closeness not only feels good, it is also good for us. Medical studies corroborate what many of us have known instinctively all along, that physical connection with those we love soothes and centers us. It also lowers blood pressure, boosts immunity, and improves our general well being. Unless the person has a cold, or might be coming down with a contagious infection, I recommend engaging in this ritual as often as feels comfortable.

So, grab a soul friend, head for the beach, the desert, a mountaintop or rooftop, to watch the sun rise or set. Cuddle and offer a prayer of gratitude. These simple things truly take care of our deeper self. And it wouldn't hurt to take along some chocolate.

CHAPTER 12

Tying Up Loose Ends:
Offerings of Love

*W*hether it looks as if your life is coming to a close or not, the topics in this chapter are worth addressing. Straightening out personal paperwork, writing or revising a will, establishing a medical directive, and resolving misunderstandings in personal relationships are important loose ends to tie up. While at first glance these may not seem to be rituals, like many things in life they hold a larger significance. All of these, in one way or another, are offerings to those you will one day leave behind. This chapter provides ideas for how you can make the process into special and meaningful rituals.

An offering is a gift that holds symbolic meaning. For example, simplifying paperwork for your family is a symbol of your love. No less than the money or possessions you leave, taking care of business in advance is a demonstration that you are continuing to care for them even after you're gone. Completing these important tasks is an expression of your gratitude for those who mean the most to you.

Also, the rituals described in this chapter are clear reminders that you do have choices. It is important to choose what you want, and then do what you can to insure that your wishes will be carried out.

A minor, but important aspect of taking care of loose ends is that once these things are done, you don't have to think about them again. Basically, once you've completed these chores you're free of worrying about them. The sense of liberation alone is worth the effort. If you should have additional ideas or requests later on, they can always be added. Crossing these things off a "To Do List" allows you to freely focus your time and energy on things that are more important—like laughing and hugging and growing.

Take care of business and put your affairs in order before your body is exhausted by disease or your life is suddenly cut short. If you wait, you may not have the time or the strength to take care of these important matters.

Resolving issues and tying up loose ends can free you to live more fully. Practice letting go of what you don't really want, or truly need, such as resentments, material things, psychological baggage, and obligations that hold no personal meaning for you. When you let go of these kinds of things, you free yourself to live more fully.

Prevent Paperwork Pandemonium

I know two men in seemingly good health who suddenly had heart attacks. One died immediately, the other survived for six days. When the latter man's wife, Deborah, opened the home safe, she found all of the important papers organized and clearly labeled. Her husband had even made funeral arrangements, so all she had to do was call the mortuary at the number listed. Deborah had not been involved with financial matters, but it was clear exactly where she stood financially and what needed to be done.

The wife of the first man, Ruth, was still in trauma months after her husband died as she searched through file boxes for records and vital papers. Even hiring a financial advisor didn't readily clarify what her financial circumstances were. It would have been difficult enough for Ruth to sort through the paperwork, but being devastated by grief made the situation seem more than she could bear, and exacerbated her sense of insecurity.

Taking care of this kind of business is not a fun task for most people, but it is an important one. If those closest to you don't thank you now for doing so, they will certainly thank you when the times comes that they need to access and understand important paperwork. If it isn't done, those left behind can feel a debilitating confusion on top of their sense of loss.

Preventing paperwork pandemonium is a great gift to those you leave behind, so let your family know where important papers are. Pulling together legal and financial papers so they are accessible and clearly marked is an offering of love. Even your closest loved ones may not know the whereabouts of these things and may not sufficiently understand them. In the shock and pain of grief, it is awful for the one left behind to feel helplessly stupid about such matters.

I know of many instances where the wife and/or children were overwhelmed trying to sort through paperwork while in a state of grief, and sometimes simply letting things slide because they couldn't deal with the financial confusion. I have seen a few cases where the family experienced great relief in discovering that everything was organized, and important documents were easy to find.

The following list will help remind you of paperwork that may be needed:

~ A written record of places you've worked and especially those where you have pensions or other benefits that might be available to your family.
~ Information on bank accounts, savings accounts, credit cards, loans.
~ Insurance policies for health, life, car, and home.

~ Tax records for at least the last three years, and preferably the last seven.

~ Investments.

~ The location of your will.

~ Title papers for your home, car, boat, or other property.

~ Armed services records if you've served in the military.

The executor for your will or trust will need most of the papers listed above.

An important note: Do *not* put important papers such as a will in a safe deposit box at the bank. The box will be sealed at the time of death and even a spouse may not be able to access the contents without a court order.

If you have always handled the household financial matters, bring someone else in on it. Turning over some of the paperwork with a full explanation to an appropriate person—spouse, adult child, sibling, or accountant—can alleviate pressure for you, and allows someone else to begin to understand what may have to be handled at some point without your input. Share with this individual your information about all the paperwork, and let him or her begin to share some of the burden of taking care of business matters. Generally, it is pretty straightforward, but consult a lawyer, accountant, or financial advisor if needed.

There is a bonus to taking care of all the paperwork. More than one person has told me, "Having done what I could to take care of those closest to me when I'm gone, has helped me to more graciously accept being taken care of by them in my illness."

One man explained it this way, "Going through these papers and organizing them for my wife was not something I enjoyed doing, but it became an act of love. I didn't want her to have to sort it out and be confused about some of it. And doing this helped me to understand that when she is taking care of me, she does it because she loves me, whether or not it's an unpleasant job. Now, I will be able to accept help from others a bit more graciously."

Sorting Through Personal Possessions

Some of us may want help, or simply a companion, as we go through boxes of personal papers, memorabilia, and other belongings. This can be a time of reflection, and deeply meaningful as you share memories connected with some of your special possessions.

Emma asked her niece, Kate, to help her go through files, boxes, and notebooks. Emma felt that Kate's presence would make the task feel less overwhelming and she wanted to be able to explain certain things to her niece. One example was a packet of letters Emma handed to Kate. "These were written by your grandfather and sent to your grandmother during World War II," Emma explained. "You'll notice that certain words or segments are blocked out. The Army read through the letters the servicemen sent home and eliminated even indirect references to where the troops were stationed or what was planned. It was a precaution. They are a part of our family history and I am entrusting them to you."

What delighted both women were all the special memories evoked as they went through the contents of boxes. "Oh, this is a letter my dad sent me when I was feeling so discouraged about my career," explained Emma as she picked up an old envelope. "It's a wonderful letter, take a look." Kate found her grandfather's words inspiring, and was pleased when Emma gave her the letter to keep. Kate was surprised to learn that her Aunt Emma had suffered such misgivings about herself when young, and this helped Kate view her own insecurities in a different light. Kate enjoyed reading a few essays Emma had written in college, and Emma enjoyed sharing the memories they provoked. Later, after Emma died, Kate counted those afternoons as some of the most special times she had with her aunt.

You might want to give away special possessions to certain people and tell the associated story, so that the meaning is passed on as well as the item. This could easily be done one-on-one or in small groups. It can be heartwarming to know that favorite possessions will have a good home and be fully appreciated. If you're not yet ready to part with a particular item, it doesn't have to actually be transferred to the recipient until later. In this case, it's a good idea to write a list of what you have given to whom, so there aren't quibbles about any of it later.

Look around your home and make a list of special things—a porcelain figurine, a box of fishing tackle, favorite books, Grandma's cookie jar—and then note next to the item the person you think would most appreciate it.

You may also want to designate a particular individual to go through your papers and possessions and determine what is to be done with them after your death. While some people wouldn't particularly care, others may see this as an important issue. It would be wise to indicate an alternate in case the first person is unable to do so for any reason.

Writing or Revising a Will

Writing a will and organizing financial papers are things that all of us should take care of long before the need arises, yet we tend to put off doing them. For one thing, we don't like thinking about "why this might be necessary." And then there is the fact that not too many of us really enjoy the actual paperwork that is involved. Still, there are reasons to push past these inner obstacles.

If you haven't written a will, do so. Whether you have a little or a lot, your assets should be dispersed the way that you want them to be. Without a will the state in which you reside will decide what happens, and the legal statutes are not always what people believe them to be. Even if you think you don't have enough assets to bother with, write a will. A written will saves your family from headaches and can help prevent misunderstandings. You can always make changes later if you want.

There are books that will guide you through drafting a will, but if your assets are sizable or your situation complex, it makes sense to consult a lawyer. First, though, think about what you want to happen and write it down—it is kind of like a reverse lottery. Be grateful that you have the opportunity to think about this and choose what feels right. You may discover that certain wishes of yours can be fulfilled in assisting others, such as helping a nephew pay for veterinary school.

You may want to write a letter stating specific things you would like the beneficiary to do, or not do, with the money being left to him or her. One of the things I learned from my husband was that the money we leave to those we love is, quite literally, our time and energy, albeit in another form. Tony felt there were particular ways he wanted his time and energy to make a difference in the lives of those he cared about. And he had very definite opinions about what he did *not* want his time and energy to support. Tony had no interest in helping people upgrade their material lifestyle. He wanted his gifts to help people grow, to help them discover life and themselves in a richer way. Since he wasn't trying to control their lives, but wanted instead to offer them a particular gift, I thought Tony's approach was one that would hold even greater meaning for the beneficiaries.

In much the same manner that people fantasize about what they'd do if they won the lottery, Tony would explore different ideas of what he thought would be beneficial for people he cared about and how he could possibly provide that. Tony refined his ideas over time, and it was obvious as he told me his thoughts about gifting money to several people close to him that this was a creative and interesting project for him.

You might want to include some added instructions or suggestions for your beneficiaries that aren't part of the legal document. For instance, "I want you to use this money to finish your education."

Or perhaps, "Take part of this money for a trip to Italy, but save the rest of it for a down payment on a house."

Maybe even, "Buy yourself flowers from me sometimes."

Your personal wishes will likely hold special meaning for those who love you.

In many cases, a simple will would suffice and it is certainly better than no will, but you might do well to take the document to an attorney to help clarify legal aspects that may ultimately save time, money, and most importantly, insure that your wishes will be honored. Writing out what you want to leave to whom and deciding upon an executor will save time when you visit an attorney. If you don't get around to the appointment, signing and dating the document will serve as a simple will. Be sure to sign it in front of two witnesses who are not beneficiaries. They must also sign and date it. (If you live in Vermont, a third witness is required.) Notarizing is not necessary.

If you already have a will, look it over and see if changes should be made. Has a beneficiary passed away? Is there someone to add? Are there further instructions? If circumstances have changed, you may want to revise your will. As an example, maybe your older brother is now a multi-millionaire and your younger sister is widowed with two boys to raise. Rather than giving each person the same amount of money, you might choose to leave the money to your sister and something of great personal meaning to your brother.

In such cases where a change is made, it is a good idea to explain to the individual(s) why you are making the changes, so they do not perceive it as a loss of affection. (Of course, if that is the reason, then it's probably better not to say anything.) It is better to explain in person, but if that feels too awkward, write a letter to be opened and read with the will.

I know of a number of cases where a wife has put off making an appointment with a lawyer, even when her husband had repeatedly requested she do so. One woman said she felt preparing for her husband's death would be accepting defeat. The reasons are generally well intended: "If we put all our energies into healing, we won't need to worry about a will. And if the treatments aren't successful, we'll deal with the will when that time comes." Generally, though, there isn't time and energy at that point to do so. Because this wife did not get a lawyer, the husband continued to worry about it from time to time until his mind became foggy. Had the details been finalized, the patient's mind would have eased and then he could have let it go.

Check your listed beneficiaries on stocks, bonds, and insurance policies. Even if your will states that everything is to go to your son, if your ex-wife is the stated beneficiary on a particular account, that money will go to her. I do know of one case where a life insurance policy had not been switched from the former to the current wife. When the ex-wife discovered this, she came forward and signed it over to the widow, saying she was sure that is what the deceased would have wanted. Rarely, though, are people quite as honorable or understanding. When death, grief, and money are combined, even individuals who would be expected to behave with kindness and compassion have stunned family and friends with their bad behavior.

Medical Directives

Specifying which medical treatments you want and don't want provides a life raft to loved ones should they be caught in a storm of medical indecision. While you may think that everyone knows what you would want, everyone may not understand it the same way. Clarifying your wishes prevents family members from years of second-guessing.

Writing down specific instructions for various medical circumstances in a legal document is termed a Living Will or Advanced Health Care Directive. Such a document, often with checkboxes, can usually be obtained through medical providers or on-line. These documents provide guidelines, but they may or may not always be adhered to—for better or for worse.

Another option is to appoint a Durable Power of Medical Attorney and this person is authorized to make medical decisions on your behalf if you are not able to do so. Discussing your wishes with your family present, including your appointed person, is wise. It will make it easier for the appointee, and for other family members, if they all understand what your wishes are.

What things do you need to look at? Most helpful would be to engage an individual who is conversant with situations that could arise. Medical providers or hospital social workers can explain possible scenarios and treatment options, along with the advantages and disadvantages of potential medical interventions. A local hospice may be able to suggest someone who understands fully what should be considered. Most hospices have booklets that explain a number of things in this regard. One such booklet, *Hard Choices for Loving People*, is available at www.hardchoices.com. A more thorough examination is contained in Virginia Morris's beautifully written book, *Talking About Death Won't Kill You.* It may be uncomfortable to look at this area, but doing so can go a long way toward providing you with the quality of life that you want should there be a time when you are not able to voice your choices.

Most importantly, you will save those closest to you from being in a state of wrenching uncertainty when they are least equipped to deal with it. Making sure your medical wishes are clearly understood can prevent family members from reproach of self and others. This is a most important offering of love to them.

Resolution of Difficult Relationships

I confess to having a fantasy about my dying. There is a family with whom I've had a strained relationship and attempts to resolve the misunderstandings have not been fruitful. Perhaps if I were dying, though, they would be fully honest and work with me to heal our connection. Maybe. And even then, maybe not. Some people can step up to the plate, and some can't. But if we have a life-threatening disease, I think we have the right to politely ask.

If it is important to you to resolve misunderstandings in your relationships with family members or friends, then it's worth making an effort to do so. But, how do you ask? How do you invite healing? Consider the following points as guidance or inspiration for taking the difficult steps to resolve old hurts:

First, define the problem clearly in your own mind without accusing others, and without justifying or defending your actions. Writing it down on paper will help clarify your thoughts and feelings, as well as bring some objectivity to the situation.

Next, write down your answers to the following questions:

What problem would you like to resolve, or re-solve?
How might a resolution come about?

What would both sides need to be willing to do?

Are you willing to do what's needed?

What would be required from the other person?

What happens when you envision a best-case scenario?

What does a worst-case scenario look like?

Are you prepared for either of these to happen?

Are you open and willing for an unexpected scenario to come out of left, or even right, field?

Whether or not you decide to contact the person, visualizations can be helpful. One possibility involves settling into a meditative state and then envisioning both of you together in a fountain with the clear water flowing over the two of you, washing away all of the hurt caused through making wrong assumptions.

Another involves envisioning a high wall that stands between you and the person with whom you have unresolved conflicts. Brick by brick, take down the wall. As you do so, become aware of the judgments that caused each of you to create this division. Continue removing bricks, and envision the other person joining you, taking down bricks from their side and participating in dismantling the wall.

One woman told me she had envisioned taking her "enemy" to a spa, and both of them had the anger pounded out of them by a Swedish masseuse. Then they sat in mud baths that drew out the toxic aspects of the relationship through their skin, and they had an herbal wrap that infused them with forgiveness. Afterward, in her visualization, they sat together in the spa dining room feeding one another a meal that deeply nourished them both. She repeated this visualization for seven nights before calling to request a conversation. While the actual encounter didn't exactly feel like a relaxing day at a spa, still, the afternoon was more productive than would have previously seemed possible.

There are those who believe we truly can invite others into a healing situation through the practice of visualization. Athletes successfully utilize visualization to improve their performance. So, it seems absolutely reasonable that we can use visualization to bring us into a sphere where we more fully embrace healing and forgiveness, and therefore, make it more likely to occur.

Once you have explored your own feelings about the situation, and have gained a clear sense of what seems possible, you may want to invite the person or persons to heal this conflict with you. Try it and see what happens. I would probably mail an invitation that said something like this:

I know I did not handle everything perfectly. I am human. I was doing the very best I knew how in very difficult circumstances.

I am sorry that something I said or did caused you pain. I would like very much to meet with you, listen to your point of view, and understand what went wrong.

It is my hope that if I understand your perspective, there might be a healing for me. I am hopeful an open and honest discussion between us might allow for healing within you as well.

Those who attempt to heal relationships generally find that something within heals during the process, even if the external relationship does not evolve to meet their heartfelt expectations. Sometimes, though, the barriers between friends or family members can fall away and leave only the sweet taste of understanding and forgiveness.

May you find that your offerings of love enrich you as well as others as you move through tying up some of your loose ends. And may completing these tasks allow you live your life more fully, and more freely.

Chapter 13

Projects

*P*rojects engage us because they offer something different from our weekly list of chores, errands, and the routine that gives shape to our days. Breaking out of that routine sometimes lends a fresh focus and a different energy to life. When Tony was involved with a project, he felt energized and had more vitality, despite the drag of chemotherapy. Thinking about his project, planning the next steps, and finding creative solutions to problems, added spice to his life even when he wasn't actually working on it. Special projects drive imagination, spark creativity, and provide a sense of completion that housework certainly doesn't give us.

The type of projects we are drawn to often change as we move from one phase to another throughout our lives. When we become aware that life does not go on forever, there may be certain projects that no longer hold interest. And there may be some completely different ones that suddenly appeal to our imaginations.

Depending on your energy level, you may not be able to tackle anything too demanding, but finding something that you relate to in your changed circumstances can provide a focus that takes you beyond your immediate situation.

This chapter offers some options that you may find intriguing, and other projects may come to you as you consider these ideas.

Whether the project is large or small, lighthearted or serious, projects helps us engage with the world in a creative manner.

Life Review

Many of us practice a form of life review on our birthday or New Year's Eve as we reflect on the previous year. Engaging in a full life review at major junctures in our lives can help us to reorient ourselves, and puts the current situation in a larger context.

There are numerous accounts of someone who thought he was about to die and reported seeing his life flash in front of his eyes—a lightning-fast form of life review. According to most religions, a life review follows death. Many people who have had a near death experience recount a life review, even among those who are not religious. Interestingly, they describe it as filled with compassion rather than judgment.

When it looks as if the end of life might be only months or years, rather than decades away, people find themselves naturally inclined to look back over their life. Most find reflecting on their experiences a worthwhile exploration. As we sift through the colorful chaos of a lifetime of experiences, we clear away dust and debris. Hidden among tangled memories, we sometimes discover precious and semi-precious stones. Uncovering these little jewels of our lives and sharing them can be a great gift to others.

Most people find that while they didn't achieve all of their goals, still, their life has held meaning and beauty. Realizing you have survived hardship and heartache, faced challenges, and offered love in many different ways can help you see the strengths you have gained, the compassion you have expressed, and how you have grown throughout your years. There are many ways to review your life, and the following ideas can help you find what will work for you.

An artist's life is often broken into phases of his or her art, such as Picasso's blue period, rose period, or cubist period. It is not only artists whose lives can be looked at in this way. Your most important work of art is the life you have lived. It can be helpful to look at events and endeavors that provide general delineations. Were the stages of your life defined by where you lived, where you worked, or by major milestones? How might you want to label these different periods of your life?

Begin by writing down names for these periods. For example, you might list school years, single and living in the city, broke and scrambling to survive, tasting success and stability, living in the duplex on Reeves Drive. Once you have identified the different phases of your life, take time to examine each one and ask yourself:

What did I learn during that phase?

What am I proud of?

What do I regret?

Whose influence was most strongly felt?

Would a color, fragrance, or perhaps a line of poetry
capture the nature of that time period?

If you could go back and relive one day of that particular period in your life, what day would it be? Try to reconstruct as much of the day as you can. Relive the sensory aspects as well as the feelings and events. Feel the cold or the warmth, be aware of the fabric of your clothes against your skin. What was the lighting like? What did you smell? After reliving that day in your mind, ask yourself if there are new things about the day you had never before considered? Write them down or tell someone.

You can take a methodical approach to life review, beginning with your birth and moving forward through each phase, or work in reverse chronological order. You could create a map on a long roll of butcher paper, illustrating the places—geographical and otherwise— that you have lived, visited, and traveled through. Or, you can simply allow memories to surface in a random way.

It is interesting to sometimes focus on one particular aspect. For example, look at the love—all the different kinds of love that were a part of the different phases of your life. Not only those who loved you, and those whom you loved, but also passions you had for ideas, songs, books, places, or hobbies. Love is, and always has been, in and around us in many guises. It is good to bask in love's varied forms and hues.

Free yourself to be creative in your approach. You might tell all the things in your life that had to do with the color orange. Or that had to do with a certain food, or a particular activity, season, or holiday. You will be amazed at the memories and meanings that are provoked.

If you are feeling stuck, or looking for an unusual approach, it might work to just be silly sometimes. Many years ago in a writing class I wrote my life story from the point of view of my feet, and included things like: "My earliest memory is dancing barefoot at my Aunt Tina's. ... My toes twinkled in the red patent leather shoes that I wore the day that.... I wore new shoes the first day of school and they made my feet feel...."

I wrote about how my feet fidgeted in church, and how my first pair of high heels marked me as a grownup, even as I struggled to keep my balance. In the process of telling the story through my feet, I discovered an entirely new perspective on my life, and loved that it highlighted details I would otherwise not have remembered.

There are many ways to engage in life review and you are free to experiment with whatever feels right for you. You might want to mix sketches, photos, and collage elements together to create a mixed media portrait of important times in your life. Simply making a list of the magical moments in your life can bring joy and healing. Many people who engage in this realize much of the magic is found in small moments. Sharing some, or all, of your life review with others can add greater meaning to the process.

Reviewing our experiences in life reminds us that we helped others bear their burdens, just as others have supported us along the way. We remember that we mastered skills, encountered greatness in the world and in ourselves. We pull out what matters from the messy and sometimes boring dailiness of life. Life review can prompt us to remember how privileged and blessed we have been. And this can help us to make peace with all we have been through.

Writing an Ethical Will

Some people find that after examining their lives, they want to pass on some of what life has taught them. This is the concept behind the ethical will, a document wherein one leaves behind one's values, one's thoughts about life and living. This is an opportunity to pass on the lessons you learned and the wisdom you gained through varied experiences.

Answering one or more questions from the following list may serve as a trigger to help you get started. And once you've begun, you may find that the process will take you where you most want and need to go.

What are the three (or five or seven) most important lessons you've learned in life?

What are three attributes you respect and admire most in other people and why?

What are the three things you are most proud of about yourself?

What are your favorite quotes, and why do you like them so much?

What are your thoughts on:

work
marriage
love
faith
parenting
money
art

If none of these questions inspire you, then write about whatever feels right. It could be computers, collecting memorabilia, teaching school, or what you learned from tending chickens.

Finally, spend some time answering the following question:

Looking at your life as a whole from your current perspective, what seems the most meaningful to you?

An ethical will can be written on paper or recorded. As with many other things, social workers and hospice centers are a good source for referrals. They may well be able to recommend someone to facilitate organizing as well as doing the actual recording.

Planning Aspects of One's Funeral

For some people, this would be too uncomfortable to even contemplate. If you are one of them, skip the next few pages. For certain people, though, planning aspects of their funeral, memorial, or Celebration of Life can be very beneficial. One woman who did so felt that it gave her a measure of control over her death—she was able to make her "finale" as creative, and decisively her, as the rest of her life had been. One gentleman took comfort in selecting a few hymns and bible passages to be included in his funeral service. Some take a lighter approach. Elizabeth Taylor, who was notoriously late for everything, stipulated that her funeral was to begin fifteen minutes after the scheduled start time.

Some might want to plan every detail, while others would offer one simple thought on what they'd like, such as stating a preference for particular flowers.

I've heard people say, "Oh, I don't want anything, don't make a fuss." If you are one of those people who does not want a funeral, remember that while the ritual would be in honor of you, it is for those left behind. A meaningful funeral can be helpful and healing for those who will need to create meaning in their lives without you. Honoring any preferences you have stated will bring greater meaning to the occasion for those who love you.

If you are not affiliated with a church, you could choose another location with special meaning. You might want to select prose or poetry to be read, or communicate what spiritual content there should be, if any.

Feel free to choose a non-traditional approach if that is in keeping with your personality. Even relatively traditional individuals might find thinking outside of the box provides the perfect solution, as did this gentleman I knew. Bert had been an avid flyer for many years, and giving up his pilot's license had been one of the most frustrating aspects of his diagnosis. One afternoon as his wife drove him past the turnoff to the small airport where he'd kept his plane, he suddenly knew just how he wanted his funeral to be. He decided an airplane hangar with all of his flying buddies present would be more appropriate for him than a church. Bert didn't want the service to be too religious, but he did want a poem read, "High Flight," written by John Gillespie Magee, who had been a pilot with the Royal Canadian Air Force during World

War II. The poem had come to be known as "The Pilot's Creed," and Bert thought it would be an apt metaphor to use.

Oh! I have slipped the surly bonds of Earth
And danced the skies on laughter-silvered wings;
Sunward I've climbed and joined the tumbling mirth of
Sun-split clouds,—and done a hundred things
You have not dreamed of wheeled and soared and swung
High in the sunlit silence. Hov'ring there,
I've chased the shouting wind along, and flung
My eager craft through footless falls of air...
Up, up the long, delirious, burning blue
I've topped the wind-swept heights with easy grace
Where never lark, nor eer eagle flew—
And, while with silent lifting mind I've trod
The high, untrespassed sanctity of space,
Put out my hand and touched the face of God.

Bert wanted his ashes to be scattered over the ocean from an airplane, and asked one of his flyer friends, Tom, if he would take Bert's wife, two grown children, and one grandchild with Tom to perform this last favor.

"You'll need to be in slow maneuverability, just above stall, so that the ashes don't fly back into the plane," explained Bert. "If my family wants to release flowers, too, that's okay with me, but I like the idea of what's left of me going from the great blue beyond into the deep blue below."

It is important to let others know what you want to happen to your body after you leave it. If you choose cremation, let that be known. Also, indicate what you would like done with your ashes.

For those who might want to plan the ceremony, there is a structural overview for planning a funeral or memorial service, along with samples, in Part Four. Also, the "Resources" section lists books that address details surrounding the funeral.

If you would like to donate your body to science, let family members know. My husband's brain was donated to brain tumor research at the hospital where he had received treatment. (See "Resources" for organizations other than a local hospital.)

Completing an Unfinished Project

Is there something you would like to finish before leaving this earth? A book, a birdhouse, the sunroom remodel? For something small, like a birdhouse, you could ask a friend or relative to help you. In some cases, it makes sense to hire someone, like the writer who hired a freelance editor to help her finish polishing a book that was close to completion.

For a large or multi-faceted project, like a room remodel, do an old-fashioned barn raising. There are undoubtedly many people who wish they could offer meaningful support. Helping you finish the sunroom would provide them with the opportunity to do so. With a half dozen handy people and an assortment of helpers, the project could likely be finished in a weekend or two. Not only will you feel a sense of completion, but inviting others to be a part of it can actually be a gift to them. In the process, you will create wonderful memories for everyone involved.

Love Letters

An extraordinarily wonderful thing to do is to write love letters expressing your appreciation and gratitude to those who mean the most to you. Many people would like to do this, but want it to be so special that they can't seem to get started. Remind yourself that a less than perfect letter is far better than no letter.

If possible, be specific when expressing your appreciation. This can make the writing easier and more interesting, and also more meaningful for the recipient. For example, writing "You are smart and good and kind and beautiful," is nice, but rather vague. The following is more specific.

"I enjoy watching you get really interested in something and then pursue learning all that you can about it from different sources. In telling me about what you discover, you have expanded my knowledge and understanding into areas I would never have gone on my own.

"I love how you always have such patience with small children, and invite their curiosity with yours.

"I love that you have your own way of doing certain things—like making, rather than buying presents for people. Or the quirky home decorating touches you create. I am even charmed by some of the things that irritate me on occasion, like checking three times that you locked the door."

The letters can include specific incidents, special memories, things said that you still hold tenderly in your heart. The recipients will cherish these letters, which is reason enough to write them.

The process of writing the letters brings with it a bit of magic. Anytime we connect strongly with love, we are graced with a touch of magic. If we spend an hour or so focusing on loving observances and memories as we write, we can bask in that luminescence for a while. And we do not walk away from the activity quite the same person who first sat down and put pen to paper.

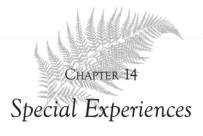

CHAPTER 14

Special Experiences

Serious illness can become all-consuming. To maintain a sense of balance, it is important to engage in activities that bring pleasure and fulfillment.

Special experiences, like projects, hold value throughout our lives because they lift us out of our everyday world for a bit. For those hours or days, we can escape the demands of daily life. Special experiences offer us a fresh perspective, and for a while, we feel freed from concerns. In addition, it feels good to have something to plan for, something to look forward to. If the things that used to be enjoyable no longer hold interest, the following ritual activities can provide a boost of energy to help you get through the more mundane times.

Story Time

Story telling is a rich tradition that has engaged people from the beginning of human history. We love telling stories, and hearing stories, whether it's a child's bedtime ritual or adults swapping stories about some event or period in their lives. Sharing stories brings us closer to one another, whether we are laughing or crying together, or simply nodding our heads in understanding.

One woman I knew who was facing a life-threatening illness, Irene, was busy working on her Life Review when it dawned on her that she had a number of stories she wanted to share. Irene was also intrigued to learn what stories others had to tell. So, she organized a group of friends and relatives to set up a Story Night every other week. Sometimes, only two people came, and at other times, a dozen or more people came to share stories. After a while, the group decided to select a theme for each night, such as:

Favorite childhood stories

Adventures large and small

Zany afternoons

Wild characters I've known

Encounters with life's mystery

Between a rock and hard place

Favorite year

Best and worst birthday

Most thankful Thanksgiving

All of those who attended gained so much from this sharing of stories that they continued the tradition long after Irene's death. It became a way for them to honor Irene, whom they missed. In so doing, the gift of Story Night continues to give to each of them, and often, they tell favorite stories about Irene.

Another family found themselves falling into sharing stories in a spontaneous way two or three times a week. It began when the father wanted to pass on certain stories to his children. Before long, they were asking for stories from when Dad was ten, when Dad and Mom met, and so forth. The children loved getting to know about their father's life before they were born. And the father inadvertently stumbled into a way of reflecting on his life that was comfortable and meaningful for him.

Make a Wish or Make a Pilgrimage

The Make A Wish Foundation was created to fulfill the dreams of children with a life-threatening medical condition, but adults benefit from doing something special, too. Fulfilling a wish inspires strength, and can rekindle belief in one's self. Such an experience enriches the lives of everyone involved with making the wish come true.

Do you have a trip or experience you have dreamt about for a long time but never fulfilled? Is there a museum or historical site you've always meant to visit? Would you love to have a few nights at a posh hotel, reconnect with an old friend, or maybe ride in a hot air balloon? What would be fun and exciting for you?

Perhaps you would like to make a pilgrimage to a special place. It doesn't have to be something grand. My father wanted to visit the ocean again before he died, so we rented a beach cottage in San Diego for a week. We checked ahead to make sure it would be handicap accessible, and we did our best to anticipate all of my dad's special needs. I made sure that if he needed emergency medical attention or supplies we would know who to call or how to get what was needed five hours from home. He enjoyed sitting by the ocean, listening to the waves, and sharing his thoughts with us.

A desired destination doesn't have to involve actually traveling. The spirit of the location or culture can be evoked through food, music, photos, and video. For instance, Michael wanted one more trip to Italy, but a physical journey wasn't possible. Michael's friends and family helped him create a virtual trip. At the party, there was a slide show of Italian locales, along with Italian food and music. The invitation included a list of common phrases in Italian, and guests had fun using words like *escusi*, *bella*, and *mangia* throughout the evening. A number of guests had also visited Italy, with or without Michael, and through sharing their stories of travels through Rome,

Florence, and the Italian countryside, they helped bring the virtual trip to life.

Sometimes, traveling can be simple. A visit to the old neighborhood can be a wonderful occasion for sharing stories and family history, as well as a time for reflection and recollection.

George visited his childhood home in a town three hours away, accompanied by his grown children and a few of his older grandkids. They had a picnic lunch in the park, and stopped by the church where he had been married. Slowly touring the town by car, George pointed out where his friends and extended family had lived, and the store where he had worked after school. They parked the car and walked around the neighborhood where George grew up. George talked about the small, yet important events of his younger life; the first day of school, the day new neighbors moved in, his first date. George even shared a few wild escapades from his youth, which gave his kids and grandkids a whole new perspective on who he was. He recalled long forgotten stories about his parents and grandparents, and found a new sense of connection with his ancestors. George's family was delighted with learning these pieces of personal and family history. They were gifts the family could pass on to future generations.

A middle-aged woman whose health was failing, Sandy, asked her sister to go with her and visit the street where they grew up. Both had driven past it on occasion over the years, but they hadn't been there together since the family moved away thirty years earlier. The sisters walked the neighborhood together and remembered, "The summers when we..." and "The winters when it was so cold, and...." They recalled the big things, the little things, the everyday things, the funny stories, the sad stories, and the interesting events. Sharing these memories brought them closer, and helped them understand how their childhoods shaped them.

Perhaps you would rather visit a non-physical place, such as a particularly happy or interesting time period that would be fun to recreate. For many baby boomers, the 1960s were an influential time that has stayed with them in profound ways. Those who danced to Glenn Miller and Sammy Kay in the 1940s recall the war and post-war years as pivotal. Recreating such a time with music, video, and memorabilia from the period can be a special experience. Look up the year or decade online and you will find an amazing array of tidbits to include on the invitation or to utilize in other ways. Let your imagination and creativity have a field day with the possibilities.

If you need some outside help to create a special experience, the "Resources" section includes a list of organizations that help grant wishes to adults, with a number of them catering to the elders of our society.

Laughter

"Laugh? At a time like this?" Absolutely! The more you laugh, the better you'll be able to handle what's thrown at you. Laughing is one of the great special experiences of life. In fact, humor is like a muscle, the more often we use it the stronger it becomes.

Numerous studies show that laughter promotes physical well-being. Laughing reduces stress, prompts relaxation, lowers blood pressure, improves breathing, and even increases muscle function.

I wanted to include a section on laughing, but wasn't sure if it really counted as a ritual. Then I looked more closely and saw that it offers much that we look for in ritual.

Laughter enhances a sense of communion. Whether we laugh with one or 100 people, we create a certain bond. Shared laughter helps cement friendships, draws us closer to family members, and can spark new connections with others.

Laughing at life's difficulties helps them seem a little less difficult, and so it becomes a symbolic slaying of the dragon of fear. Laughing at life's bizarre changes helps us feel we can handle them. Laughter helps us regain balance by putting things in perspective—sometimes by exaggerating them out of all proportion. Laughing with someone else at our crazy thoughts and feelings helps us feel a little less crazy. And laughter helps us transition out of fear and anxiety, into a frame of mind that we can cope, and so we feel stronger.

You can watch funny movies and stand-up comedians that bring you into their cockeyed world and make you laugh. Invite friends for a potluck meal and request that they bring a funny story to share. Laugh at the absurdity of life's situations and the ridiculous predicaments this world sometimes presents.

Laughing at the ironies of life helped Tony and me get through our ordeals. We laughed at things daily, especially when we were in the hospital. Laughing helped us get through all of it, drew us closer, and helped us keep our sanity. Our laughter was counterbalance to the seriousness of his illness, and the grind of medical treatments.

Norman Cousins, who was the renowned editor of the *Saturday Review* for many years, was also an author perhaps best known for his book, *Anatomy of an Illness.* Diagnosed with a "rare and incurable disease," Cousins recovered from his disease and lived decades longer than his doctors predicted. He attributed much of his longevity to his commitment to laughter as a form of healing. He once explained, "I made the joyous discovery that 10 minutes of genuine belly laughter had an anesthetic effect."

Western medicine is doubtful about laughter's ability to fully heal serious illness, but medical studies have verified that laughter improves the flow of oxygen throughout the body. One study showed that "patients who watched funny videos during certain painful procedures were more relaxed and tolerated the pain longer. It also found that cancer patients had less pain and slept better after such entertainment." At the very least, laughter can do no harm, and can certainly help you feel better.

My mother serves as a testament to the power of laughter. She has little regard for germs, while I am finicky about them. At 87, she is stronger and healthier than I am. I think it is due in part to the fact that she laughs easily and often. Like love, faith, and hope, laughter is a wondrous experience. Laughter may or may not help you live longer, but it will certainly help you live better.

Rituals to Invite Healing

There are a number of variations on this ritual, such as prayer circles, chanting, and working with visualizations. We can invite healing into our lives by opening ourselves to the stars in the sky, to a higher power or a divine force. And we can open ourselves to the healing power within.

Having a connection with a deity helps many people feel they are not alone, and they have support in their healing. Some people surrender to a sense of harmony in the universe, drawing metaphoric connections between the spiral of galaxies spinning through space and the spiral of DNA within each and every cell in the body.

All of us have a number of individuals who have helped us heal along our path through life, be they friends, family, teachers, or those in the healing professions. Draw upon all sources of healing, including the love of others, and love of self.

Healing the body is important, but other aspects of us may also need healing. There are two important questions you might want to consider:

What do I need to heal before I can fully live?

What do I need to heal before I can die in peace?

You may want to ponder these questions aloud, or explore them in meditation. You could also experiment with "free writing," which is a process where you keep your writing hand moving across the paper without stopping, allowing the words to flow from your pen without thinking about what you will write next. This method helps keep the critical mind from impeding spontaneous insights.

I have led group healing rituals where a few people or as many as twenty gathered to focus on healing. If you would like to do something like this, I have included the following ritual as an example. Select an appropriate person to lead it, and make whatever changes you want to the script. You could also pull sections of this ritual to use in meditations or visualizations.

Robert and his wife, Lynne, wanted to invite special friends and family to offer healing support to Robert as he battled his cancer.

The family sent an invitation that read:

On Sunday evening, some of Robert's family and friends will gather at his home for a circle of healing. While the primary focus will be on inviting healing for Robert on all levels, we want to extend the energy of healing to all of those in attendance.

Think of one area in your own life that wants healing. Bring a symbol of this, or write it on a piece of paper.

Also, please bring three free-standing candles, such as pillar candles. We will begin arriving at 7:30, but please arrive no later than 8:00. Dessert and coffee will follow.

About a dozen guests attended Robert's Circle of Healing in his home. They all sat in a circle in the living room with a central table to hold the candles. Once everyone was seated, Robert's wife, Lynne, dimmed the lights in the living room, indicating the beginning of the ritual. (Keep in mind that you can adapt the phrasing to suit your circumstances and beliefs.)

On behalf of Robert and Lynne, I thank you for coming. I don't know of anyone on this planet who isn't in need of healing in some area of life. It seems that a part of being human is the need to constantly heal our bodies, our minds, our hearts, and our spirits, too.

It is also part of being human to want to be healed, and to want to help in someone else's healing. Just as it requires love and compassion to want to heal another, love and compassion toward ourselves are necessary for our own healing.

[Lighting Robert's central candle.] We invite the spirit of love and compassion into our midst. May we each feel this spirit glowing in our hearts as we focus on the flame.

As the light burns stronger, let it radiate all the way through you. Then release it to flow out from you, directed back toward this flame. May the light from the flame then reflect it back onto each one of you, its strength amplified.

Lynne, will you please lift your central candle and light it from Robert's, so that this light of love and compassion can be passed around the circle. Steve, will you tilt your candle into Lynne's to take that light and then pass it on.

As each of you takes the light and passes it on, the light grows within and around us. As the light of love and compassion grows brighter in the room, let it grow stronger within each of us.

Let love flow forth from your hearts, and allow it to flow freely through your veins and arteries, filling the body with love for its being.

Let the love fill your lungs, and then breathe it out into the world. Every breath in, take in love from the world around you. Every breath out, feed the world around you with your love.

Let us now focus the love and its healing on Robert. Breathe in from the vast reservoir of love and compassion that has shined upon this earth since time began. As you slowly exhale, let that love flow forth to Robert. [Allow for several breaths.]

With love and compassion filling our circle, we now invite the spirit of healing. [Lighting Robert's right candle from his central candle.]

An underlying aspect of healing is to pinpoint the area of discord, then bring it into a state of balance and harmony. As you focus on this flame, feel your body coming into a state of balance; allow all of the different functions to ease into a comfortable place of harmony. Also allow this to happen in regard to any areas of your life where there is discord. [Allow a moment.]

Lynne, please light your right candle from Robert's. As we pass the light of healing, come to understand that healing helps you to feel whole, and feeling whole helps in your healing. Feel yourselves healing into truth, [Pause] healing into kindness, [Pause] and healing into harmony.

Bring the light of healing into yourselves. Feel it healing your wounds, healing the pain of past hurts, healing any discord within your body, your mind, your heart. Allow it to heal your spirit, and let that bring healing to all of the cells and synapses, healing to the blood. Let it bring the functioning of all the organs and glands into balance and harmony with one another.

Allow the light of healing to bring body, mind, and spirit into a state of deep and profound ease.

Now let the healing go beyond yourself and focus this healing energy on Robert; inviting ever greater healing into his body. Invite healing into his psyche. [Pause] Invite healing into his deepest heart. Focus now on inviting healing for the spirit [Pause] and for the spirit to assist in healing all the cells in his body.

Invite healing in all its forms to help in healing all that can be healed. We invite this healing to grace Robert and all of those present.

Lynne, if you would light your third candle and then place your symbol at its base. Name the healing that you invite in.

Lynne: "I invite healing for strained relationships with family members. And I invite great healing for Robert."

[The next person then lit his third candle from his central candle, placed his symbol on the table, and invited healing for his issue and for Robert. Moving around the circle, each person followed suit, inviting healing for his or her issue and for Robert. Then...]

Please join hands, and then close your eyes. Feel the energy of deep healing coming up through the soles of your feet, and flowing through you, filling your heart. Feel your heart adding love to that healing energy.

Send this energy out through your right hand and release it to flow around the circle. Accept that energy coming into your left hand. Let it flow through your body, healing all of you as it passes through you and then out your right hand as it continues on around the circle.

Allow yourself to bask in this energy; let it grow stronger as it moves around and through the circle. Know that this healing energy is there for all of us to tap into, and know that it always grows stronger when it is shared.

[Pause, allow people to experience the healing energy before proceeding.]

Let the movement of the energy around the circle slow, and feel it growing even stronger the more slowly it moves. As it gradually comes to a stop, let it fill you completely—body, soul, heart and mind. Feel each cell and synapse pulsing with that healing energy. Allow the energy that you have invited into yourself to rest within you.

Releasing hands, reach out to take your symbol and hold it close. Send the energy into your symbol. Feel the healing process beginning. Feel it being sent out beyond this moment to continue the healing as you move through the coming days and weeks.

Now, closing our eyes again, let us take another moment to focus our love and healing on Robert. Feel it flowing from you into him, and may he allow that healing love to penetrate deeply. [Pause to take several breaths.]

Opening your eyes, please push your central candle to the center of the table as a symbol of the healing energy you have brought to Robert, and will leave with him.

Robert, lift your right candle, a symbol of the healing energy you have passed on, and offer it as a gift to Lynne. Lynne, please offer your right candle to the person on your right. Continue around the circle, accepting the candle from the person on your left as symbol of the healing energy you receive from others.

Your remaining candle you will keep, as a symbol of the energy of healing you have invited into yourself.

To close, let us take a moment within ourselves to offer gratitude for the spirit of healing. Recall times when you were healed, and give thanks for each one.

[Pause for a few minutes to give people time to reflect.]

Thank you all for joining in this healing. As we open the circle, let love and compassion and healing flow out into the world.

When Tony was in the midst of his cancer treatment, I organized a similar ritual. We found that the love and affection our friends expressed was healing for Tony on many levels. After that special gathering, Tony opened up more, and despite the limitations of his illness, I watched him blossom. Like a plant that's been recently fed, something deep within Tony was nourished in that healing circle. Though Tony's cancer didn't go into remission, something deep within was healed, and that was an important healing for him.

I witnessed a simple, but very effective version of a healing circle at a birthday party for Clark, a man in his late fifties who was likely celebrating his last birthday. In this case, the ritual was spontaneous and brief. A musician friend was a guest at the party and entertained for a while, playing his guitar and singing. At one point, he put down his guitar and asked those gathered to join him in a prayer. He asked for healing for Clark, for strength, for love, and for peace. It took only a few minutes, but it was enough for Clark to feel the love and support of his circle of friends gathered there in his living room.

Chapter 15

Remission or Recovery

$\mathcal{P}$atients move through the ups and downs of the journey through treatment hoping to hear the words "recovery" or "remission" from the doctor. They invest their precious time and energy in working toward this goal. They undergo all kinds of procedures and treatments believing they will recover their health. They look forward to the day when the doctor walks into the examination room with a smile saying, "I have good news." There is joy and a great sense of relief upon hearing these words. But, like so many other things in life, there are generally additional thoughts and feelings that can sit side-by-side with the feelings of relief and happiness. The flow often goes something like this:

Given a reprieve!

Released from the medical treatment routine!

Free to go back to "Normal Life!"

I got another chance! I get to have more life!

All of these thoughts, and more, are possible. Then comes the sudden realization that you will go back to "normal life" as a changed person.

This transition can catch people off guard. One would anticipate that there would be relief and a sense of celebration, and usually there is. Sometimes, though, there are a number of unexpected feelings: depression, fear, guilt, anxiety, disappointment, sadness, or grief. It is not at all abnormal to experience these. It is possible to be incredibly grateful that you are one of the lucky ones, and still grieve certain losses. It is even normal to miss going for treatment, either because of bonds formed with medical caregivers or because now you will have to create a new structure for life and don't know where to start.

It is helpful to pay attention to all of the thoughts and feelings, and make an effort to understand them. Talking it through with a friend or counselor who is open and accepting of the full kaleidoscope of feelings can be very helpful, and is generally more therapeutic than trying to deny emotions that you may judge as out of place with the good news.

A Ritual for Reorienting Back to Health

Some patients feel guilty that they survived their illness and not someone else they knew. In a different way than at diagnosis, there is the question, "Why me?"

And the answer perhaps is found in asking other questions, "What can I do with this, as the person I am now? What feels right to do?"

You will need to regain your balance and reorient yourself once again. The rituals in Chapter 4, "Reorienting," can support you in this process. The following ritual can also be helpful if done thoughtfully and with a sense of purpose.

Undoubtedly, there are objects that have accumulated that relate to your illness and treatment. Gather them together into four piles.

1. Things that can now be disposed of.

2. Items that might be needed later if there's a recurrence.

3. Articles that are reminders of people's love and caring.

4. Objects symbolic of changes that have occurred.

If there is an empty pile, find something to serve as a symbol. Now, take time to really look at each object in the first pile. Pick up an object, hold it, think about what it means on its own. Also, what is the larger thing that it symbolizes? Perhaps one of the items is a bottle of anti-nausea pills. The immediate meaning is that the pills helped you tolerate the side effects of chemo. The larger symbolism is that of generally feeling sick. Now, your body is stronger and healthier, you can throw those pills away.

Take time to regard each item in the first pile. Let it sink in fully that you are able to let go of those things now. Then ceremonially take the items to the trash, or recycle them, freeing yourself from what they represent.

Spend time with the second pile. If you were to have a recurrence, how would these items help you? What do you know now that would allow you to better move through that experience? Think about your fears connected with recurrence. What can you do to better protect yourself from that possibility? Resolve to do what you can, and do your best to accept that some things are beyond your control.

Put the items into a box, then put your fears in the box as well. Close the lid, and put the box away somewhere. Anytime you are having anxiety about your health, if there's nothing that you can actually do, mentally consign the fear to this box.

The third pile holds mementos of those who care about you. Take time now and allow yourself to bask in their love and affection. In the future, they may not express it as intensively as when you were ill, but know that their love and appreciation for you is still strong. Accept that these people need to turn some of that attention back to their own lives now, but don't forget how much they went out of their way to offer support when it was most needed.

Place these symbols of love and affection in a grouping, or in places scattered around your home, as reminders of how much people care about you. Never forget how special it was to have them be there for you. Feel supported in knowing that these people can be counted on. Before long, see if there are at least small ways that you can be there for them. Write thank you notes to some of the people who supported and helped you in your healing. You might even select a small gift for some people, a symbol for them of how much you care, and how much their caring means to you. These are ways of deeply connecting with the web of caring that surrounds us all.

The fourth pile may take a little longer, and you may need to find some additional objects to serve as symbols for ways in which you have changed. This can be challenging, but also most interesting. Think about the ways in which you could, and could not, step right back into old patterns of the old life.

What needs to be different now?

How can you use what you've learned to be better in your job, with friends and family, with setting priorities and keeping them?

What new elements do you want to add to old activities, whether work, chores, or pleasure?

What now is needed for you to move forward with an open mind and trusting heart?

Place these items on an altar or in a special place. But first look at them closely. Try to more fully understand these changes, what they mean to you, and how they will affect this new phase of your life. If there are other changes not reflected in these objects, find objects that will serve as symbols.

Write down or discuss with someone close to you what will be important as you create a new structure for your days and weeks. What aspects of your changed self do you want reflected or expressed? Periodically, spend time contemplating these symbols as you move forward on the next segment of your life journey.

A Map for Family and Friends

Chapter 16

Suggestions for Using Part Three

$\mathcal{W}$hen someone we care about has a serious illness, we often feel helpless. We want to fix it, but there isn't anything we can do to magically heal the person. This doesn't mean, though, that we can't offer meaningful help. The chapters in Part Three can help ease this sense of helplessness by providing an understanding of patient needs, along with suggestions of what can be done to offer support.

The nurturing presence of family and friends can do so much to assist patients in healing through their illness, and if need be, living as fully as possible all the way through their dying process.

Serving as an Escort

When the doctor told us Tony had a brain tumor and would need immediate surgery, we felt blindsided. Though my life was impacted as much as his, still, it was Tony who would be wheeled into the operating room the next day, so I forced myself to stay focused on the doctor's instructions of all that we had to do before then. I knew I needed to deal with the practical matters so Tony could try to absorb the enormity of what was happening to him.

Then, and in all the months that followed, this was a call to higher service. The people around us also answered that call, each in different ways. Tony and I were deeply grateful for the love and sensitivity many people showed us, and we struggled to understand the behavior of certain others. All I could fathom then, and even now, many years later, is that those who were close and didn't do much to help didn't understand what they could do, were too uncomfortable to offer, or didn't see the importance of demonstrating support through their actions. Discomfort at being not quite sure how to behave can sometimes prevent individuals from offering the help they want to give.

The chapters in Part Three provide insight into the patient's journey, along with direct guidance, allowing primary caregivers, family, and friends to feel more comfortable being present and offering support.

If the disease goes into remission or the patient recovers, understanding and emotional support will be appreciated as he or she makes that transition. If the patient's journey leads toward the end of life, helping him or her to live meaningfully through the passages is an amazing and life-expanding experience for both giver and receiver.

While family and friends can fight certain battles for the patient, like pushing through the bureaucracy of insurance companies or intricacies of the medical realm, the patient is fighting the major battle on a daily basis. Primarily, caregivers can stand behind or beside the patient and serve as escorts to smooth the way and offer support.

I have witnessed rituals of initiation where the person being initiated is blindfolded. During this time, an escort stands on either side to offer assistance through the process. A patient moving through the wake of diagnosis, critical periods, or final passages of life, is much like that blindfolded initiate. The patient, like the initiate, has an inner sense of things, but cannot see what exactly is coming or what will be experienced. It is helpful and comforting to have respectful escorts.

To serve as an escort, you must be willing to move past any preconceptions, your own discomfort, and especially, your own point of view, in order to honor the patient's needs and values. In this service, if you continually practice the courage of an open mind and open heart, you will grow in ways you could never have predicted.

As an escort, if you are respectful, honest and kind, you will experience deep sharing and, believe it or not, a new and deeper sense of joy. You will also learn some things about the mystery of life through encountering some of the mysteries of facing death.

The rituals in Part Three offer specific suggestions as to how friends and family can provide better support for the patient. If you are fortunate, the patient will have noted some of his or her preferences in the following chapters and this will provide guidance for you. If not, use your best judgment as to what you think will be the most appropriate and supportive for the person you are attending. Not what you would want, not what you think the patient should want, but what your best and most compassionate judgment says that he or she would want under the circumstances. An excellent book, *20 Things Cancer Patients Want You to Know* by Lisa Whitlow, provides insight into what can be most helpful, or most irritating to patients.

While Part Three focuses primarily on helping friends and family offer meaningful support to the patient, it also addresses some of their own needs during such difficult and confusing times.

Looking over the rituals, you will acquire a better understanding of what to expect, and how you can participate in the patient's process. I encourage you to offer support in a multitude of ways, and do your best to follow his or her lead.

Following the Patient's Lead

People don't always say straight out what they want or need, so it is important to look for clues, and ask questions that provide an opening. "How are things going?" often provides a more comfortable opening than "How are you?"

If the patient talks about the illness, follow that thread. If he or she changes course, follow. Do your best to stay open, and listen with care. You don't have to have answers, you need only be willing to try and understand what it is the patient is experiencing.

Perhaps you can help the individual find his own answers by asking questions. You might ask:

What are your choices?

What do you see as the pros and cons of these alternatives?

How do you feel about that?

How are you dealing with it?

How do you want to be handling it?

Open-ended questions such as these can lead to meaningful conversations that may help you better understand how to offer emotional support and practical help.

Sometimes, following the patient's lead happens in a more subtle way, as illustrated in the following example. Patricia, a bright and artistic woman in her early sixties, talked with me about her elderly mother who was nearing the end of life. "Mom's body is getting weaker, but she keeps holding on," Patricia explained. "Lately, she's been acting like she's only about three years old. I know she can still feed herself, but she won't eat unless I feed her."

Patricia was obviously disconcerted by her mother's regression. I theorized that perhaps her mother, Alice, was feeling like she was three years old because she was as vulnerable and dependent as a small child. I also offered that perhaps early childhood had been a pleasant time in Alice's life and she wanted to return to it.

Patricia responded, "No, that wasn't at all a happy period. Her family was going through difficult changes and she had been sort of pushed off to the sidelines."

In response, I suggested that maybe Alice needed to have that time period healed. "For whatever reason, that's where she needs to go, so follow her lead," I encouraged. "Try treating your mom as if she is the most adorable three year old you've ever encountered."

A month later Patricia called and told me she had followed my suggestion and it had made a world of difference. "Once I stopped being frustrated and impatient, suddenly Mom was delighted by almost everything. Much of the time it was truly delightful to be around her. It was a completely different kind of relationship, but Mom and I enjoyed one another more than we had for years. A week ago, as I was feeding her some oatmeal for dinner—the only thing I could get her to eat—she gently pushed my hand away and said, 'I've had enough now.' She died peacefully the next morning."

Working with Prayer and Meditation

Generally, the rituals in this book are spiritually inclusive, meaning they do not address themselves to any particular religious point of view. The spiritual aspect of these rituals can be easily changed to provide a better fit for the patient by adding, altering, or deleting spiritual aspects.

Because widely divergent views on religion exist in our culture—sometimes even within the same family—spiritually inclusive prayers and meditations are offered throughout.

The following are some simple ways to shift the wording of prayers or meditations, from this book or other sources, so they more accurately reflect the beliefs of the patient.

For example, the basic idea of "Dear God, give us strength to ..." can be rendered to "May we find strength to ...." And of course, the reverse can be done.

The following basic sentiment can be expressed through three different points of view.

Religious: May God, the divine source of love, surround and support you.

Spiritual: May the source of all love surround and support you.

Non-spiritual: May you feel our love surrounding and supporting you.

Feel free to cross out anything that doesn't feel right in a prayer, make changes, and add what seems needed.

Sometimes, there will be just one phrase that provokes a strong connection. Take that phrase and use it in whatever ways seem appropriate. You might repeat it over and over in a mantra, and then allow other thoughts and words to come in and become part of the mantra. Let the process unfold until it becomes a prayer from your heart and spirit.

As an example, there were two lines in a prayer for end of life written by an author of spiritual books, Starhawk, that struck a chord in me.

You go from love into love.
Carry with you only love.

I have used these lines in any number of different ways. I have quoted them in conversation, offered them as the basis for a melodic chant, and as a meditation exercise. I have spoken the words softly in prayer and allowed them to attract other ideas and words. I have used these lines at a patient's bedside, helping the patient to focus first on all the love that surrounds him or her here, then on all the love that is beyond, naming the love the patient will move toward—whether deity or loved ones who have passed on.

Let your mind and spirit work freely with what holds meaning, and seems appropriate for the patient.

Patients need support from family and friends throughout their journey, especially in the first few months following diagnosis, anytime there is a crisis or transition, as well as when a patient is nearing the end of life.

The following chapter, "Aftermath of Diagnosis," offers suggestions on how friends and family can offer meaningful support to the patient and the primary caregiver, along with some guidelines for things to say, and some things not to say. Even if you are reading this book late in the patient's journey, I suggest you look over the next chapter to gain a general understanding of the special needs of patients.

You can then turn straight to the chapter that addresses the passage that the patient is currently passing through. If you have time, take a look at the chapters before and after that one. You may see something of value you can use in the current situation.

CHAPTER 17

Aftermath of Diagnosis

*B*efore Tony was released from the hospital following his initial brain surgery, the nurse showed me how to dress the surgical wound and explained Tony's medication schedule. The nurse provided me with a basic understanding of how to handle the seizures Tony would likely have. We were given an appointment to meet with the radiologist the following week so Tony could start radiation treatment. Aside from that, we weren't given any information on how to live in this radically altered life.

We were fortunate to have Moray as our close friend. She had a key to our apartment and had cleaned our place, washed laundry, and stocked the refrigerator while I was staying with Tony at the hospital. With so many new, and previously unimagined things to suddenly deal with, it was an enormous gift to have household chores taken care of for us.

The time following diagnosis often seems surreal for patients and family members. They are struggling to absorb the news, regain their balance, and comprehend the medical world so they can understand options for treatment. The shock waves keep reverberating through minds and hearts, and impact every aspect of life.

Friends, extended family, and co-workers are also impacted, often feeling helpless in the face of such terrible news. While they usually are helpless in terms of providing a cure, there is much they can do to help the patient in a variety of meaningful ways.

Emotional Support and Practical Help

Our friend Moray seemed to know instinctively just what Tony and I needed, and she never seemed uncomfortable around us. Many of Tony's male friends, though, seemed ill at ease with his new vulnerability. I thought perhaps sharing an activity might help the men move past the discomfort, so, Tony began suggesting an errand to run when male friends visited. A trip to the hardware store could sometimes result in the two men working on a small project together. Those who entered into activities with Tony more easily moved into being comfortable with him in his changed circumstances.

Diagnosis of serious illness creates a huge shift in the patient's life, and those close to the patient are also affected. They may be spurred to action like our friend Moray, but often they feel confused and helpless. Having a sense of what they might do to offer meaningful help can combat those feelings. The following suggestions may help you see ways you can offer support.

Bring Food

One time-honored ritual is to bring food. It not only provides practical support, but also nourishes on deeper levels. Be sure to check on dietary restrictions and preferences, and strictly honor them. If the patient is eating only organic foods, or doesn't eat meat, or gluten, or dairy, it is important to follow the stated guidelines—even if the patient occasionally breaks these food rules, or is gracious when offered non-organic grapes.

If needed, friends, neighbors, and co-workers can organize a food brigade. A "captain" coordinates a schedule, and volunteers deliver meals to the house two to five nights each week. Depending on the size of the brigade, and how often meals are needed, each person may only need to bring dinner once or twice a month. A free, on-line service, Mealtrain.com, is a wonderful community tool that greatly simplifies coordinating food deliveries.

Such practical help is greatly appreciated, but the loving support that is expressed through generous acts is even more important. Providing food is not only nourishing, but also nurturing, and offers sustenance emotionally as well as physically. Small wonder that the ritual of bringing food during difficult times has been practiced century after century in cultures all over the world.

Tony and I had a couple of people who took turns preparing organic meals once a week and delivering them to us at dinnertime. Though we often invited them to stay and eat with us, they rarely accepted. They understood Tony and I needed downtime together. While we did enjoy their company, we were most grateful for their sensitivity, and we could taste the love in the meals they prepared, even in the leftovers we enjoyed a night or two later!

Support in Action

Demonstrate your caring. Supportive actions lift the weight of practical burdens, symbolize the affection and concern that you feel, and help to lift the patient's spirit. Your emotional support is manifested in your actions.

Often, people will say, "Let me know if I can help."

It is better to ask, "What can I do to help?" and check in regularly, asking this same question.

Don't just ask once and then figure they don't need anything because you never heard from them. Gently be persistent. You can also be more specific by asking, "Can I go to the market for you? Run an errand?"

When you visit, look around, and listen for clues of what to offer. During a period when Tony and I didn't have a washing machine,

Moray came by on Friday each week after she got off work, gathered up our dirty laundry and brought it back on Monday, washed and folded. She was a godsend! Others noticed that an electric shaver would be simpler for Tony, and that we could use a juicer. We hadn't had time to even think about these things, but were grateful when the shaver and juicer were offered as gifts.

If you are a bit of a handyman, offer to help with something around the house, such as repairs or minor improvements. If nothing needs attention at the moment, you could say, "If you ever do need anything, please don't hesitate to call me. I'd love to be able to help in some way."

If you are not a very good cook, but reliable, offer to organize a phone tree. It was incredibly helpful for me to have only two phone calls to make at critical junctures so I could give Tony's care my full attention. One call was to a member of Tony's family, who then passed the information to the rest of his family. The other call was to Moray, who had a list of names and numbers of those who needed to be informed. In turn, some of those individuals passed on the information to others who needed to be in the loop. Moray knew to alert the women who brought meals: "Tony is in the hospital, so hold off on the dinner. I'll let you know when he's going to be released as I'm sure dinner would be most welcome then."

If you're computer savvy, you could be a tremendous help. Perhaps the patient needs some research done on the internet, or needs help straightening out a software problem. Maybe you are the one who organizes a group email.

Neighbors can be especially helpful because of their close proximity. Offer to pick up prescriptions or groceries in a pinch, take out the trash cans for weekly pick-up, mow the lawn, or walk the dog. All these thoughtful acts would be of greater help than you might imagine.

Perhaps you could help with grocery shopping. During our initial adjustment period, Moray took it upon herself to do the grocery shopping for us. Later, whenever we were in a crunch period, Moray stepped up. Having one person willing to somewhat regularly do the marketing can be a tremendous help. This means the patient or caregiver doesn't have to explain that "milk" means a half gallon of two percent organic milk, or if the asparagus isn't organic get broccoli instead. If the grocery list can be e-mailed, it's easier still.

If you have a flexible schedule, you could offer to take the patient to treatments or doctor appointments.

During times when the patient needs a lot of care, offer to visit with the patient for a few hours while the caregiver runs errands, or takes a much needed break to visit a friend, see a movie, or get a haircut.

Strapped for time, but have some money? The ritual aspect still applies. Sending a gift card for a masseuse to provide massages at home for both patient and caregiver is a ritual offering of rejuvenation. Arranging for someone to clean the house periodically gifts the couple with extra time together. Taking the patient and caregiver out for a special night on the town is a ritual reminder that they are special people who deserve a special experience.

Your intent alone can turn an activity into a ritual. I frequently gave Tony a foot massage, and sometimes I made it into a ritual by adding the intent that this would enable him to feel a stronger connection to the earth. As I massaged Tony's feet, I visualized him being grounded firmly to life and all its unexpected variables. The symbolism lent a different focus to the activity, and also created a more powerful energy connection between us.

Tony usually enjoyed visitors, but was most appreciative of those who demonstrated their caring by actively participating in his life. Through freely offering support in many of the previously mentioned ways, they participated in his healing.

Don't let awkwardness deprive you of the opportunity to show your love and support during such an important time. Interestingly, those who did the most to help Tony later told me they grew in unexpected ways from sharing in our experience, and were greatly enriched through developing a greater closeness with Tony.

Helping the Primary Caregiver

All of those who offer help and support to the patient in any number of capacities are caregivers, but the word usually refers to the primary caregiver.

In the wake of a diagnosis, the primary caregiver is experiencing many of the same stressors and feelings as the patient. Shock, anger, fear, or disbelief can cause the caregiver to be as disoriented and overwhelmed as the patient. Yet, the primary caregiver needs to stay grounded in order to support and take care of his or her loved one. Caregiver is a demanding role that requires strengths heretofore untapped, and no one can do it all without help from others.

Moray did so many things for Tony and me during his illness that sometimes I felt awkward accepting so much help from her. I was especially uncomfortable with Moray's generosity when these thoughtful things were for me rather than Tony. One time I talked with Moray about this, and she explained, "There's only so much that I can do for Tony directly. But if I do things to help you, then you have more time to do the things that only you can do for him.

Because there is so much that only you can do, my helping you is one of the ways in which I can help Tony the most."

To this day, I send Moray my gratitude and my blessings.

Honor Patient's Values

Be very mindful of this, especially in those areas where the patient's values are different from your own. In the magical realm of myth and fairy tale, a circle drawn around an individual can provide protection against negative forces. Imagine there is such a magical circle around the patient—one that even protects him or her from your good intentions.

Do not impose your beliefs about diet, doctors, or the mind/body connection. Especially, do not impose your spiritual beliefs. You may say, "My faith has supported me in my difficulties. If you would ever like to talk about it, please let me know."

Say only this and only once. After that, leave it to the patient to initiate any further conversation about it.

If the patient chooses to pursue a spiritual discussion, regardless of your own beliefs, remain open to understanding the patient's point of view. It is important not to impose our beliefs on someone else, first and foremost out of respect. But I have also learned that if we allow a patient to formulate his or her own thoughts about death, we can sometimes gain additional insight.

I am particularly grateful for a conversation I had with one patient, Claire, who told me she thought a phrase we often think of as a euphemism is actually a more accurate description of death. She explained, "When people say 'passed on' rather than 'died,' they are closer to the truth, or what I see as the truth. When we die, we pass on from this form of existence into whatever comes next. Maybe it's kind of like passing from fourth grade into fifth. Maybe it's more like graduating from college and going out into the wider world.

"I don't know what it will be exactly—I can only sense it in broad metaphors," Claire added. "I just know that in passing away from this world, I will pass into another. Matter and energy cannot be created or destroyed, they simply change form." Claire's perception of the phrase "to pass on" shifted and enlarged my sense of context.

If the patient should open the door to a discussion of your spiritual beliefs, be alert for any signs that say, "I've had enough for now."

This same approach holds for other suggestions you may have such as, "This regimen cured my neighbor's sister," and any other topic on which the patient doesn't share your passion or point of view.

Honor Patient's Need to Conserve Energy

In the days following chemo or hospital stays, a patient usually will require more rest. The first few rounds of chemotherapy might be well tolerated, but the fifth one might knock the patient flat for a week or more. Be mindful that the patient's time and energy are limited, and know that priorities will shift from time to time.

If the patient doesn't give you a sense of his or her needs, then check with the primary caregiver to get a better sense of the patient's energy level.

In general, keep groups of visitors small. Sometimes the patient is up for a party, but there are times when even three family members can feel like a crowd, requiring too much energy.

Take the lead from the patient, and also check with the caregiver. Sometimes, the patient will say something is okay when it really isn't because he is hesitant to appear sick, weak, or ungracious.

Respect Patient's Choices

When there is a lot going on for the patient, it can feel overwhelming. His or her body is weakened and the individual may not have the usual level of confidence. Be particularly conscientious about supporting the patient in his choices. If his choices seem less than wise to you, you may ask, "What led you to this choice?"

Then, keep an open mind and truly try to understand it from the patient's point of view. You may gently put forth your opinion, but then leave it alone. Do not take advantage of the patient's vulnerability to push your values. Remember the magic circle I mentioned previously? Use it here.

Be aware that even though something may seem crystal clear to you standing on the outside, no matter how close you are, you cannot know the fullness of what it is to live in the circumstances of the patient. Your assumptions may not be correct, and it would be unfair to cause additional difficulties based on your misapprehensions.

Tony and I were always careful to honor one another in our relationship, but I became even more vigilant about this after his diagnosis. There were others, though, who seemed to feel it was okay to push their opinions on Tony, and question Tony's decisions about any number of things. Though they were well intentioned, Tony was angry with them for not respecting his judgment. Even if the patient's choices are not the ones you would make, respect the patient's right to choose, and support him or her in those choices.

Also, keep your negativity about others to yourself. A few weeks after Tony's diagnosis, he related to me an incident earlier that day with his friend, David. I felt that David not only failed to exhibit any compassion, but was somewhat taking advantage of Tony. I became angry and indignantly expressed my opinion of David's actions. In the midst of my outburst, I saw a hurt look on Tony's face, and suddenly realized I was basically saying David wasn't being a friend to Tony. My intention had been to defend Tony, but in effect, I was saying David didn't care about Tony. I stopped my tirade, and was careful after that to never criticize anyone else's behavior toward Tony.

If Tony was critical of others, which happened on occasion, I would simply listen. After he vented for a while, I would remind him of other things the person had done to be helpful, assuring Tony that this person did care about him even if the behavior didn't always reflect it.

Being supportive means being careful not to undermine the patient, even unintentionally. One patient I worked with, Craig, found himself in an emotional landmine near the end of his life. Craig's mother, Helen, had liked his fiancé, Fran—until Craig got sick, and then her opinion changed. Helen thought Fran was only offering care and help to Craig in order to get his money. When Helen voiced her opinion to Craig, he really didn't believe that was who Fran was, but it planted a poisonous seed of doubt.

When Craig's hospice volunteer told me about this, she voiced her suspicion that it was Helen who had ulterior motives. "His mom visits once a week, brings in food from one of her—not his—favorite restaurants, and never offers any practical help. Craig's friends offer more help than his mother does. Fran is there almost 24/7, and so loving in how she takes care of Craig—you couldn't buy that kind of care."

The hospice worker paused for a moment, then added, "I know I'm not supposed to get involved with something like this, but I'm so tempted to tell Craig that I think his mom is not only totally wrong about Fran, but that Helen is probably the one after his money."

After hearing her story, I cautioned the hospice volunteer, "Saying such a thing could undermine Craig's relationship with his mother. Not only is it not your place to say anything about it, but relations with family are important. Accusing Helen might cause Craig to feel that even his mother doesn't really love him. You don't want that."

A family counselor who was present added, "It's possible that Helen has a misplaced sense of wanting to protect her son. She can't protect him from the cancer, so that energy may have gone into trying to protect him from something else—even if she's wrong about the threat. Perhaps, since Helen isn't willing to do all that's required to care for her son on a daily basis, Fran's behavior seems suspicious in her eyes."

The counselor offered this advice, "Do all you can to reinforce to Craig the love you see between him and Fran. Ask about their history together. As Craig talks about it, he will likely be reminded of how much both of them have been there for one another over their years together. But do not say anything negative about Helen."

The counselor's compassion and loving approach were exemplary in this sticky situation. She suggested to the hospice volunteer, "You might try to understand Helen better. Perhaps she feels as if she isn't needed, or important in her son's life. She may not put herself out in the way that others do, but that doesn't mean she doesn't care about her son. If there's an opportunity, let Helen know of something she might do that would be appreciated. You could also try to counter Helen's insecurity by telling her that she holds an important place in Craig's life."

Over the years, I have found this is not a unique situation. Surprisingly, it is often the accuser who does the least to help. No matter what your relationship to the patient, be careful about ever accusing someone of helping the patient for ulterior reasons. It can impact the patient very badly, undermining his sense of self-worth. Helen didn't realize that what she was saying to Craig was, in effect, no one would want him for himself now that he was ill. Unfortunately, that was how Craig took it. Take care that your actions and words support the patient.

Even when doing our utmost to be sensitive to a patient's feelings, miscommunication can create difficulties. Listen carefully, and ask for clarification when it is needed. It can also be helpful to have a family member or counselor talk with the patient and find out about pet peeves and desires, then pass the information on to others. Remember, what might be most welcome for one patient, could be the last thing another patient wants. Each person is different, and needs and wants sometimes change when illness alters the landscape of life.

CHAPTER 18

When Bedfast for Brief or Extended Times

$\mathcal{M}$ost of us have had the experience of being impacted enough by illness or injury to be bedfast for at least a while. When our capacity to go out and actively participate in the world is lessened, we usually welcome visitors who bring the world to us. Unless we are terribly ill, we appreciate the love they bring, the stories they share and their desire to hear our stories—including our complaints!

When we are physically weak, we are necessarily in a place where we receive more than we are able to give. At these times, life asks us to be open, and receptive.

Remembering our own experiences of being physically weak can provide a small sense of what the patient may be feeling, and help us reset our expectations. Each one of us responds to being dependent in our own way, and we all have our own particular difficulties with adjusting to such a circumstance. Be patient with the patient.

The following rituals are simple and provide a way to offer love and affection to your friend or family member who is confined to bed. Many of us feel more comfortable if we have something to do; we feel a little less helpless. While the value of practical support cannot be overestimated, your open and receptive presence is also a gift.

The Gift of Your Presence

When visiting a friend or family member who is bedfast, it is often helpful to take a few moments before entering the patient's home or room to breathe and let go of any worries or discomforts you may have. Take a few slow, deep breaths and open yourself to being fully present with the person who is ill, wherever he or she may be emotionally at that time. The patient may be full of wit or full of despair; be willing to meet in the moment, whatever the mood might be.

Sometimes, when we're ill we don't want to be cheered up. Sometimes, we simply want someone to be with us where we are, able to accept whatever our frame of mind might be. We usually want someone willing to listen, and willing to talk about what we feel like discussing.

Visitors need to leave all preconceptions outside the patient's room and enter with an open mind and heart in order to better perceive the needs and wants of the patient. Listen without judgment, without trying to fix what can't be fixed, while at the same time being open to creative solutions for improving what could be better.

Listen carefully. Ask thoughtful questions. You aren't expected to have answers to everything. When asked, offer your thoughts, and then hand it back to the patient by asking, "What do you think?"

Ask to hear the patient's stories—the present and the past. And if you're not sure where to start, it might be appropriate to ask, "What would you truly like to talk about today?"

Bring Gifts of the World

When you visit a friend or family member who is bedfast, consider bringing a gift that provides a connection to the natural world; perhaps an interesting plant, a quartz crystal, a seashell, or a beautiful rock. Such gifts can be particularly valuable if the patient is in an impersonal setting such as a hospital.

Flowers are often appreciated, but it is best to avoid strongly scented blooms, which can be overwhelming in a small or closed room. Be aware that patients going through chemotherapy are often particularly sensitive to strong odors.

Enhance the Environment

Creating a pleasant environment for someone who is bedfast is an offering of love. There are simple things to notice: Is it possible for the patient to have a more pleasing view? If the view can't be improved, provide a landscape painting or photograph. If possible, bring in a few choices and ask which one would be most welcome in his or her line of vision.

Perhaps the lighting in the room would be better if it weren't so bright and harsh, or is the room too dim? If the patient is at home, it's generally a simple matter of changing light bulbs. And it's relatively simple to install a dimmer switch, which provides more control of the lighting level. You might check to see if the sheets and blankets are soft. A warm throw in the patient's favorite color would be a lovely gift. The following are some other gift suggestions.

Fragrance

Fresh branches of pine or rosemary in a vase can bring a lovely natural scent into a room, and the rich green brings the world of nature to the bedside. Lavender is also lovely, fresh or dried. It is usually best, though, to check on the person's preferences since some people may have an allergy or aversion to certain fragrances.

Most people find the scent of lavender calming, and lavender water or oil is soothing to the skin. Lavender water can be sprayed or sprinkled on the pillow, or on the person's neck and arms. Lavender oil might be rubbed on the temples or wrists. A bowl of lavender buds is a wonderful gift. Reaching into the bowl and crushing the buds to release their fragrance can become a tiny relaxation ritual for caregivers as well as patients, particularly when combined with a few slow, deep breaths.

Generally, it is best to use natural aromas rather than synthetic scents or perfumes. If fresh isn't available, use essential oils subtly since they are concentrated.

Avoid scented candles, and in most cases, incense. Both can be overpowering for someone who is not feeling well, and the smoke from the incense usually isn't good for someone who is ill. (Keep in mind there are those for whom the ritual burning of incense is connected with their faith tradition, so honor the patient's choice.)

Candles

The soft glow of candlelight creates a special atmosphere of warmth and intimacy. Sometimes, candles are lit to begin a ritual, and then blown out at the conclusion.

CAUTION: **If oxygen or other flammables are present, avoid all flames, including incense.** Other concerns when using candles include the following:

~ Be aware that candles produce heat and use up oxygen, so don't overdo it.

~ If you do use candles, use caution. Do not place them too near the bed where they could be knocked over.

~ It is best to use pure beeswax candles, which don't release toxic byproducts.

~ Be aware that candles and incense are generally forbidden in hospitals, and in many convalescent centers, for important safety reasons. Check with a representative of the facility before striking a match.

Music

Playing music some of the time can be calming and provide respite from words, allowing thoughts to flow, sometimes tears, or private prayers.

In general, peaceful and soothing music seems best—classical music, perhaps Gregorian, Buddhist, or Native American chants. Some patients would enjoy the family singing favorite songs or hymns, others might prefer listening to the Beatles. Perhaps the patient would welcome the recitation of favorite poems. Think in terms of the patient's preferences, and ask if he or she would like something in particular.

For someone in a hospital, a CD with continuous play can bring ocean waves, rain, or nature sounds throughout the night to soothe the patient when sleep is elusive, or to provide a calming white noise to muffle hospital sounds.

It is good practice to check with the person who is ill, rather than assuming something will be soothing. Even if the patient seems not to be conscious, try to gauge the effect of the music. Is the patient calmer or more agitated? And be aware that what may be right at one time may not be later on.

Don't forget the music of silence, which allows for the bird's song and the rustle of leaves to be heard.

Saying Magic Words

It can be especially important to say the magic words: "I love you," and "Thank you." Even if you have said these things previously, they can certainly be said again. Saying, "I love you" and "Thank you" can be repeated at different times in different ways. I don't think we can say, or hear, those magic words too often at any time of life.

Whether it is done with a formal gathering, or casually one-on-one, there are many ways to say "Thank you" and "I love you." One way to do so is to tell the person, "This is what I've learned from you...." Then offer specific things the person did or said that taught you valuable lessons or provided you with insight.

The following are two examples of gatherings that focused on expressing appreciation for the patient.

When Gail's brother Greg became bedfast, she didn't want him becoming discouraged. She asked if she could come by one evening and bring a half dozen of Greg's friends. The group sat around Greg's bed and each person thanked Greg for something special he'd done for them. Then each friend told Greg something of value they'd learned from him over the years. While some of the evening was serious, there was also much laughter and teasing of one another.

Afterward, Greg's wife said, "All those friends telling Greg that his life and who he is, and what he's said and done, held meaning for them, was so incredibly meaningful for Greg. It was a form of life review through the eyes of his friends."

While bedfast, Greg's thoughts about his life had been focused on what he hadn't done. It was amazingly helpful for him to be reminded by his friends of important ways that he had made a difference in their lives. Most of the incidents Greg's friends mentioned, he'd forgotten about, or didn't think were any big deal. Greg's wife observed, "There has been a really important change in Greg since then. He's reclaimed a sense of self-worth that had been eroding. I am so grateful to Gail and all of the guys!"

A similar ritual involved an exchange of flowers. Alison had done well with the early stages of chemotherapy, but as she neared the end of the scheduled treatments, her body and spirit were worn down.

Her mother asked me to create a ritual that would help strengthen her spirit.

Seven of Alison's friends each brought several stems of flowers that were placed in a special vase as they each told her "Thank you" and shared an important way in which Alison had helped them to blossom in their lives.

Then, over a special catered lunch at the house, Alison and her friends shared more stories about how they had inspired and supported one another. After Alison's friends left, the bouquet of lilies, roses, lilacs and peonies served as a reminder of the love and appreciation each person had expressed. Despite her deep fatigue from chemo, Alison felt a new sense of gratitude blossoming within her.

When we tell someone pieces of the story of his or her life from our vantage point, we offer a form of life review that often sheds a completely new light on that person's sense of self. I have done this in bits and pieces with an elderly aunt in recent years as we've reminisced together. A friend of mine drew an outline of his father's life and told his father's story from a son's perspective as a gift to his dad. The father was awed that his son had learned important lessons from observing him over the years, as well as from the lessons he'd consciously tried to teach his son. It confirmed for this father that he had not only lived a meaningful life, but that he had been a better father than he thought.

Appreciation and gratitude shared from the heart can be simple and powerful. Even casually telling the patient about something he or she did that impressed you, can be deeply meaningful.

Turn Patient Care into Caring Rituals

Sometimes ritual evolves out of practicality. After Tony's second surgery, he was bedfast for about two weeks, and had only minimal mobility for another three weeks. During this time, I began washing his face and hands at night, and this quickly grew into a ritual. I would wet the washcloth with warm water to make it more relaxing, unless it was hot out and then I'd use cool water. I would massage his face as I washed, focusing gentle pressure on his temples, the jaw hinges just below his ears, his mouth, and sinus areas. I repeated this three times.

The first time, my focus was on washing away the stresses of the day and releasing tension. Then, after rinsing out the washcloth and warming it again, the second time I focused on sending my love for Tony into my hands so that it would flow straight into his body. The third time, my focus was on channeling my love and Divine Love through my fingertips. I hoped that in some way the power of this loving energy might penetrate through skin and skull and help to heal the tumor growing in his brain. For the final part of our nightly ritual, I would wet the washcloth one more time and massage Tony's hands, treating each finger with caring attention.

It is difficult to explain why, but there was such sweet intimacy in this, so we continued the practice even after Tony was out of bed and could care for himself. For me, the "magic three" was part of what made it into a ritual, along with the intent connected with my actions. Tony lived far longer than the doctors had predicted, so perhaps the ritual influenced his healing, though I will never know for sure. I do know with certainty that Tony felt the love and caring expressed through this ritual, and I loved sharing this interlude with him.

If the patient is bedfast for an extended period of time, providing a bed bath will be most welcomed. Nurses or hospice can explain the technique, or you can do an Internet search for "giving a bed bath" and find complete instructions, some with video.

Your intent can bring this, or any activity, into the realm of ritual, and you can augment the ritual aspect by using special basins or towels. Adding a pleasant fragrance, lighting candles, or simply talking lovingly to the patient can enhance the experience. Consider what might be special or meaningful for your loved one, and incorporate that into the ritual you create.

Adding a symbolic component to an ordinary action can turn it into a simple but meaningful ritual. Shampooing hair, shaving, cleaning dentures, and rubbing backs are all caring activities that could become loving rituals. In addition, they are generally most welcomed and appreciated.

Even something not so pleasant, such as changing a colostomy bag, can become a caring ritual. If you have trouble with this idea, consider the following perspective when changing a bag. You could even say this aloud: "Because of this bag, you are still here. I am glad to do this because I love you, and love having you with me."

Something like this not only turns the chore into an offering of gratitude, but can also help the patient feel more comfortable having you take care of it.

CHAPTER 19

Holding Vigil in the Final Days

$\mathcal{A}$s for all major rites of passage, some preparation or instruction is necessary for those offering love and assistance at the end of life. There may be medical or practical things you need to know about, so ask your doctor, nurse, or hospice worker for any specific instructions. Generally, though, there really isn't much to do except offer comfort, love, and a supportive presence.

During the final days, family and close friends will often sit in vigil with the patient. The term vigil means "to be awake and attentive, observe and protect." Early usage involved spiritual observances on the eve of a holy day—and dying is a holy time. Understanding some general guidelines can help you feel more comfortable in your vigil with the patient.

While circumstances will vary depending on the illness and the individual, generally, in the final days the patient sometimes will not seem conscious, yet at other times will be alert and clear. The patient may or may not be aware that he is near death. If the patient says something about dying, do not contradict him—you may be depriving him of the conversation he most wants, or perhaps needs. Give him space to talk, and respect what he says. Ask questions that will help him clarify his thoughts and feelings. I used to think I needed to have answers, but I now understand that listening attentively is more important.

If the patient asks, "Am I dying?", tell him what the doctor said, then ask, "What do you think?" Patients often know their own bodies better than the doctors do.

If the patient says, "I'm afraid to die," you can ask, "What is it that scares you?" Sometimes, it is the final dying process itself that causes apprehension. You can reassure the patient that all living things seem to know exactly what to do when the time comes, and he or she will, too. You might add that while we may have known nothing about how to be born, and despite difficulties in that process, we made our way into this world just fine. (The end of Chapter Ten provides a description of the dying process, which may be helpful to review.)

Sometimes, patients are afraid of what comes after the dying. None of us knows for certain, but those who have clinically died and been revived generally describe the experience as wonderful, beautiful beyond description. One woman described her brief experience of death as being surrounded by a profound radiance, and feeling that radiance flowing within her as well.

Sometimes, a dying person is concerned about an unresolved issue or piece of business. You can explore this concern with him or her and see if anything can be done to address it in some way.

Perhaps the patient has a particular need or desire. Asking questions can help identify what is needed. If the patient is distressed, try to understand what it's about—there may be something that can be done to help. Look over the rituals in Part Two: A Map of Patient Choices, perhaps something there will provide insight into what the patient needs.

Be aware that patients nearing death will sometimes use symbolism, almost like dream images, to communicate, and this requires an open and creative way of listening. A common metaphor involves travel, and the patient may seem incoherent, insistent on finding a ticket or passport. In such a case, you might provide a facsimile ticket and explain it will take her wherever she wants and needs to go.

Even an actual passport might not work for another patient who insists, "I need the *real* passport." You might ask what that passport looks like, how it is different, and what this real passport can do that the other one can't. The response may provide a clue as to how you might offer comfort and calm the patient's concern.

Family and friends who hold vigil at a loved one's bedside do what can be done to help ease the passing. Be aware that a mindful, loving presence is most important. As a person moves closer to death, he or she needs to feel supported and loved. He or she also needs to be helped to let go with love. The following rituals provide ways for friends and family to meet these needs.

Offerings of Love and Support

When I had visited Uncle Ray the day before Thanksgiving, he was sitting in a chair and we had a long conversation. When I returned to see him again three days after the holiday, he was no longer conscious. My connection with him went back as far as I could remember; now, suddenly it seemed there was no way for me to connect with him. I stood there with my hand on his and told him I loved him. I thanked him for taking the time to talk with me when I was little and everyone else always seemed too busy.

I didn't know if he heard me or not, there was no change of expression. Studying his face, hoping for some response, I noticed his lips were dry, so I asked my aunt if I could give him some water. She said the doctor had told her that he shouldn't be given anything to drink, but it would be okay if I swabbed his lips or fed him a small amount of ice chips. As I slowly fed my uncle the slivers of ice, I began to relax. This simple act of tending to his needs gave me a way to connect with him, and a way to express my love.

Do simple, caring things such as swabbing a dry mouth, or wiping the brow, perhaps with lavender scented water. These practical and comforting acts fulfill a number of needs: the patient's need to feel loved, the need of others to connect with the person who is dying, and a way to demonstrate love for him or her.

Touch is usually appropriate: soothing caresses, holding hands, gently placing your hand on their arm or heart. The warmth of our attentive presence is a gift, even if no words are spoken.

It is very important to listen carefully when the patient does talk. Take what is said seriously, even if it doesn't seem to make sense. Remember, it makes sense to the person who is dying, and it may make sense to others later on.

The morning of my father's last day he told my mom, "They're going to make me over."

Humoring him, she responded, "That's good, then you won't hurt anymore."

He thought for a moment, then said, "They're going to make me over *completely*—electric, I think.... Yeah, all electric."

When my mom later told me about this, I suggested maybe he was talking about becoming pure energy, maybe he had some real sense of what was going to happen to him. Mom responded, "I thought he was kind of out of it like he had been the last several days. Maybe he was connecting with what would happen to him, or where he was going." Then she added, "Oh, I wish I'd asked him more questions about it."

We don't truly know what is occurring in the psyche of any individual as he or she approaches death, but we shouldn't dismiss a dying person's comments or perceptions simply because we don't understand.

My dad hadn't been fully responsive since shortly after the "electric" comment at breakfast, nevertheless, when I was leaving the hospital that night I told him, "Daddy, I'll see you tomorrow."

Surprising all of us, my dad responded, "No, not tomorrow."

While his response was unexpected, we didn't think the comment was anything more than him echoing my last word. My dad died two hours after I left. Then, I knew that he knew—"Not tomorrow."

Communion

Rituals connected with a patient's religion can be especially meaningful in the final days. They might be end-of-life rituals, such as Last Rites, and might include Confession or Communion. Clergy are usually willing to come to the bedside for this. Close friends and family might also want to take part.

Roger's elderly mother, Ruth, had been ill for some time when the visiting nurse called to tell him his mother probably had only a few days. Roger arranged for Ruth's pastor to visit, offer Communion, and lead them all in prayer. The pastor also invited the family to tell Ruth how much they cared about her. There were tears as well as laughter as Roger, his wife, and their two daughters shared their feelings and special memories with Ruth. She went to sleep that night with a smile on her face. Amazingly, over the next few days Ruth's health began to improve and then, she managed an almost complete recovery. Ruth greatly enjoyed the next six months and then, one night died peacefully in her sleep.

People sometimes avoid these "last rites" rituals, fearing they will hasten death somehow. Not only is that an irrational fear, but one that can prevent a meaningful experience. A last communion ritual does not often coincide with remission, but can still provide a powerful healing influence.

Communion is a particularly versatile ritual that occurs in many traditions. One example is the Christian Eucharist in which the bread and wine are consecrated then shared with those gathered. In Judaism, there is the saying of Kiddush when the wine is poured for the Sabbath meal. In these and other traditions, the purpose of the ritual is to connect people with one another, as well as bring the focus of the group to the holiness of life. The communion ritual affirms connection with what is transcendent, and with what helps us to transcend.

Those not affiliated with an organized religion can draw upon the basic concept of the communion ritual and create their own version. This is what Christina and her family did when her sister, Abbie, was dying.

The family cleaned Abbie's room in preparation for the ritual. They gently bathed Abbie and washed her hair. Christina brought a vase of flowers, along with seven candles that she lit and placed around the room. A friend had been to Ireland and brought back some water from a holy well.

Christina began the ritual by pouring the holy water into a special chalice. She lifted the cup in salute to her sister then told Abbie about the different ways she had helped and inspired her. Then Christina handed the chalice to her father who expressed his love for his daughter as he shared some of his favorite memories. The chalice moved from one to the next, each person holding it as they spoke of their love for Abbie.

When the chalice had completed its round, Christina offered the chalice to Abbie who drank from it, taking in all the love and gratitude each person had expressed. Years later, Christina still cherishes the memory of her sister that day, thin and frail, yet glowing. Christina said it was as if she could literally see all of their love reflected back at them through Abbie's eyes.

Co-meditation

This ritual can be particularly helpful during nonresponsive times when we feel a loss of connection with a patient. This was particularly difficult for me when my dad was dying, and I wish I'd known to do something like this. With my husband, it was something I did instinctively on a number of occasions when Tony was sedated or in a crisis, and when he was losing consciousness toward the end of his life. Only later did I learn there is a name for this connection—it is called "co-meditation," and it is a common practice in some cultures.

To co-meditate, simply sit in silence breathing in rhythm with the other person. Open yourself to being fully present with him. Don't try to imagine what he is thinking or feeling, just breathe in rhythm with him.

In Buddhist tradition, one enters into union with another through this practice. But you don't have to be Buddhist or even have meditated before. Just allow your body and mind to become quiet as you inhale and exhale in unison with the patient. Allow the breath to be enough, the only thing you need to do or focus upon.

As your body and mind grow calm, listen to what is being breathed at the still center. Allow the sense of connection to be felt without trying to make it do or be anything other than just what it is. Simply open yourself, and breathe in unison. Let yourself connect through the heart, through the breath.

A Litany of Gratitude and Love

It is generally believed that people retain their sense of hearing until the very end of life, so continue talking to the person even after he or she has become nonresponsive. The patient may or may not comprehend the words you say, but will certainly sense your warmth and affection. It is not unusual for people who have been non-responsive for some time to suddenly respond to something said to them, so always assume that what you are saying will be heard on some level.

If you are uncertain about what to say, you could offer a wandering list of those things for which you are grateful, randomly interwoven with the things you especially love about the individual. I did this with my husband one night toward the end of his life, even though he was no longer responsive. I carefully slipped under the tubes and wires to cuddle with him in the hospital bed. As I held Tony, I told him how glad and grateful I was that he had come into my life. So many moments from our years together came flooding in, and I shared my reminiscences with him. I told him how much I had learned from him, and how grateful I was for all of the wonderful memories of our time together.

"I remember that day at the beach when.... The Thanksgiving we spent just the two of us.... The first time you hugged me, and how right it felt to have your arms around me ...."

Several days after Tony died, I recalled this and was so glad our last conversation was spent sharing my gratitude and sweet memories with him.

A number of years later, I sat at the bedside of my favorite aunt a week before she died and offered her a long, loving list of gratitude and appreciation for all she had done for me. She was awake and listened carefully. It was heartwarming to remind us both of the special connection we had shared for over fifty years.

Prayers for Letting Go

In many cultures and religious traditions, people pray at the bedside of the dying to assist in lifting and guiding the spirit to move toward God, Allah, Yahweh, "the Godness," or the patient's personal conception of a higher power. Affirming and honoring the spiritual beliefs of the person who is dying offers comfort and support, as well as providing a sense of purpose, a sense of direction even.

Some have a strong faith to which they turn for prayer. For others, prayer isn't at all appropriate. Some who don't usually pray, but have spiritual beliefs, might be grateful for something simple.

Please note that whatever your own beliefs, it is most important that you honor the beliefs of the person who is dying. This is not the time to take advantage of the patient's vulnerability and press your spiritual point of view. While the Baptist sister and Catholic brother may have argued religion over the years, this is a time to work from common ground and honor the dying person's preferences.

It is not uncommon for there to be a range of beliefs in the family to be taken into account, so the prayers that I offer in this book are generally spiritually inclusive. The following draws upon a tradition from the Quakers that holds great beauty and meaning in its simplicity:

Gather in community and hold one another in the Light.

That's all there is to it. Simply hold one another in the light. You can use this basic idea and build a ritual around it to provide some structure if desired. The following example creates space for prayer, without promoting any particular spiritual or religious beliefs.

Please gather in a circle around Chris and take the hand of the person on either side of you.

Through Chris, we are all connected to one another. In joining hands, we create a circle of love to surround her.

Closing our eyes, let us focus on holding Chris in the light. [Hold for a moment or two.]

Let us hope that she feels fully the love that radiates from our hearts.

Let us breathe slowly, deeply, as we hold her in the light of all love.

In a few moments of silence, let us each in our own way offer a prayer of love for Chris.

Squeeze hands to send the love around this circle, and may Chris feel it all around her.

May the love always move around and between us all. Amen.

Another prayer speaks directly to the one who is dying:

> Envision yourself floating free of this earth,
> weightless of all worries,
> peaceful in wonder
> as your spirit ascends into a pure and radiant joy;
> the soul's heart free to give a greater light,
> and free to receive an even greater love.
> We pause now to be still,
> to breathe in gratitude
> for all the many blessings of love.
> Thank you, [name], for being you,
> and for the great and deep privilege of knowing you.
> May your spirit shine in grace, now and forever. Amen.

Even when honoring an atheist point of view, a circle to hold the patient in the light of love is certainly appropriate. Richard knew that his parents would want to pray at his bedside when he was dying. Being an atheist, he wasn't at all comfortable with that scenario, so I created an "atheist prayer" for him that stated his boundaries without negating other points of view.

Religious prayer would not be compatible with Richard's values, but we can gather here with reverence for human life, and the human spirit.

We can allow the power and beauty of the human spirit to uplift us all.

May this help us to accept that the entrance and exit to life are veiled in mystery and wonder.

May the power of love remind us that the beauty of the heart lives on, echoing and shimmering through many other hearts.

May this spirit of love allow us to shine in gratitude for the gift of Richard in our lives, and may this grateful shining uplift Richard's heart and spirit.

May the light of compassion give us strength to be fully present, and aware of how we may best offer help and loving support.

Before closing, we pause for a moment to breathe slowly and deeply, holding all of us in the light of love.

Saying Goodbye

One of the great regrets with sudden death is that we do not get the opportunity to say goodbye and to tell the person one last time, "I love you." As hard as it is to say the last goodbye, it is a time for which we should also be grateful.

We sometimes avoid saying goodbye, afraid that it may make us cry. But even if it also makes the one who is dying cry, those tears need to flow, and they are a sign of love.

A way into saying goodbye could begin: "I will miss you when you go. I am so glad that so much of you has become a part of me."

Then move into saying whatever feels right to say.

If you need a way to close this, you might say: "I love you, you will always live in my heart."

Or, "I will always remember our friendship, and I am glad that you are a part of who I am."

Just before dusk on my father's last day, the family gathered around his bed. Though he was no longer responsive, we told him how much we loved him. We told him he had done a fine job with his life. My siblings and I thanked him for giving us life, and expressed our appreciation for the gift of having him to father us through the years.

We all told him we would miss him, but it was okay for him to let go of the struggle for life. We told him we would be okay, and that we would all take care of one another. And we promised to take good care of Mom for him.

We said goodbye, and we kissed him. Then we hugged one another and cried. It was painfully sad, but it also felt right. The experience was healing for everyone in our family.

It may seem odd, but sometimes patients need to be given permission to die, for any number of reasons. They may hold on for longer than is comfortable thinking that those being left behind aren't ready or able to let go. Or they may have concerns about those they are leaving. Reassuring the dying person can allow him or her to move away from this life more easily, less encumbered by worry.

My husband had the ability to tell me what he was thinking, and what he needed even after he wasn't fully coherent. Five or six days before Tony died, he said to me with some urgency, "I need brave."

I reassured him that he had brave. "You have fought so hard, so well for so long now. You had the courage to face this disease and its complications and continually rise to meet the challenges. You are so very brave! I trust that you have the courage to face anything you need to."

After that, I would tell Tony several times a day how brave he was, and remind him of how much courage he had demonstrated in his life.

A few days later he whispered, "I don't know if I can fight anymore, it's too hard."

I moved closer and put my arms around him. "You can stop fighting and let go whenever you need or want to. I will miss you! I have so loved having you in my life, but whenever you need to go, it's okay."

Then I whispered, "Do you want to let go now?"

"No," he answered, "not yet."

I breathed a sigh of relief. "Oh, good. I want you here with me as long as possible. But when you need to go, it will be okay to let go. I love you, and I will miss you, but I will be okay."

Tony nodded in understanding.

The patient doesn't always provide such an opening, so the family or someone else may need to create a circumstance that provides a way into giving permission to go.

You may want to invite those present to gather in a circle and visualize holding the patient and one another in the light. You could also use a prayer or meditation to help bring a sense of the spiritual into this time.

Simple and conversational also works. You might say, "You seem to have difficulty breathing. If that becomes too much of a struggle, it's okay to let go. It isn't being weak to accept that you are too tired to continue fighting."

The most important elements are reminding the dying person of his or her worth, and expressing how much he or she is loved.

CHAPTER 20

Near the Time of Passing

The first time I was present when someone died I was awed by the simplicity. My Uncle Ray breathed in, there was a long pause as if time was suspended, and then slowly, he exhaled. He lingered for several seconds in the space between. He took another breath, gently let go of the breath, and then, he simply did not breathe in again.

It was so quiet and peaceful the moment might have slipped past without being noticed, except that something enormous had happened. Some part of him that had been there just half a moment earlier was gone. Uncle Ray's body was there, but Uncle Ray was not.

To witness this splitting off of energy and matter, the magical coming together of which translates into a life, is as awe inspiring as birth. However it is phrased—body and soul, flesh and spirit, matter and energy—they each release their hold on the other. At the same time, for just a moment or two, there is a sense of wholeness, a sense of completion and completeness. I felt privileged to be present at my uncle's death. Several hours later, I realized, "This man who taught me so much about life when I was little, as his parting gift, he taught me about dying." Stunning that something so enormous, so profound, could be so simple, so quiet.

The actual moments of the passing are brief, yet profound beyond description. A reverence for the moments of leave-taking seems built into us. If we understand a few basic guidelines, our natural instincts will help us know what we are to do. A nurse, or another member of the patient's care team, can give you some idea of what you might expect. It can be difficult to ask the questions, but having answers reduces confusion and uncertainty, which will allow you to be more present.

Of course, it is an emotional time, but try to keep in mind that the focus needs to be on the comfort of the dying person. As much as possible, strive for a peaceful, calm, and soothing atmosphere. With your loving presence, offer care and support, serving as a midwife to the passage. Like birth, death comes in its own time and on its own terms.

It seems that individuals sometimes choose to die when no one is present. A friend shared with me a not uncommon story. "Someone had been with my dad twenty-four hours a day for over a week. One evening, the entire family went to the hospital coffee shop for a break. We were only gone fifteen minutes. My dad died while we were away."

I have heard so many stories of people dying "the one time that no one was with them" that I now believe it is by design. It may be that some people need to die alone, and for any number of reasons cannot let go when others are present. So, even after Tony became nonresponsive, I always told him where I was going, and how long I'd be gone. I wanted him to know so he could choose whether he wanted to leave his body while I was out of the room, or wait until my return.

An individual will sometimes wait until someone close arrives from out of town. "Hang on, Mama, Joey's coming." Sometimes Mama needs to see Joey, and sometimes she doesn't. There may not be a need for a last encounter because everything is resolved, or Mamma knows that Joey will be fine.

Sometimes, a patient will hold onto life until after a particular date or event. I know a number of people who died within the first few days after Christmas. To some extent, it does seem we choose when to let go of life. Even though not fully conscious, my father's last romantic gesture was to honor his wedding anniversary on May 2 by spending it with his wife. He died shortly after midnight on May 3.

Individuals nearing death will sometimes behave as if they see someone others do not. They may hold out their arms or say the name of someone close who has previously passed on. Sometimes in a final burst of energy, a patient will get out of bed to move toward something only he or she can see. Generally, the dying person is comforted by these presences so it shouldn't be cause for alarm. Whether you feel there is a certain reality to these events, or that the person is merely hallucinating, will depend on your own beliefs. Many hospice nurses, and others working in end of life care, have witnessed a number of these occurrences, and they believe there is something other than end-stage hallucination involved.

While we cannot orchestrate the patient's dying, there are rituals that can help us support someone in the dying process. Mostly, what is required of us is to be warm and loving, open, and as fully present as possible.

Surround the Patient with Love

When someone is preparing to let go, we do not want to hold him or her back with our love, but instead, hold them up with our love. Those present could:

~ Create a circle of love in silence.
~ Pray or chant according to the beliefs of the person who is dying.

~ Co-meditate. (See Chapter 19)

~ Listen to the patient's favorite music or sing. Some hospitals and hospice centers can arrange for a harpist to come to the patient's room.

The following ritual is simple and can be easily altered or elaborated upon.

People stand around the bed with their fingertips just under the person's body, and say together:

> With love in our hands,
> we hold you up with love.
> With love in our hearts,
> we help to lift you free with love.

Allow space for silence, prayer, or for people to speak from the heart, then repeat the lines to end the ritual.

The lines could be said by each person present one at a time, or chanted by everyone. It could be done with one person reading the line and then others repeating. The lines could also be said by each individual as he or she arrives at the bedside or leaves it.

One family of singers sang the first two lines in rounds, their voices blending in spontaneous harmonies. Each then took a turn singing his or her love and blessings. They closed with singing the third line a number of times before moving on to the last line, letting their voices soar before then falling into hushed tones as they sang "amen" at the end.

The spirit of this ritual could also be manifested without saying a word. A young woman I worked with, Tess, liked this ritual and regretted that her mom and sister wouldn't be open to it. While Tess did not want to impose her values on her family, she very much wanted to bring a spiritual dimension into her father's dying for herself. Tess was able to do so without causing her family discomfort. She quietly stood by her father's bed with her fingertips resting under him, and focused intently upon the lines in the prayer, sending her energy and loving support to her dad through her hands and her heart.

Lifting the Spirit with Love and Blessings

This ritual can be done as is, or used as a template from which you can draw thoughts and phrases to use in a more spontaneous and unstructured way.

Stand around the bed with fingertips just under the patient. One person stands at the foot of the bed and reads each line, others stand on either side of the bed and repeat the words:

Our love surrounds you.
  Our love supports you.
    We thank you for being a part of our lives.

Our love surrounds you.
  Our love supports you.
    Our love serves to help lift you free.

When the light calls you,
  the light is yours to go to.
    The light is yours to lift you into joy.

Our love surrounds you.
Our love supports you.
When you are ready, breathe free.

(Use the following three lines only if it is in keeping with the patient's
beliefs, or is altered to be appropriate.)

God's love supports you.
When you are ready,
breathe yourself into his arms.

Let yourself flow into radiance.
Our love will go with you.
Our love will always be with you.

Our love surrounds you.
Our love supports you.
Our love will go with you.

Our love will always be with you.
Our love will always be with you.
Our love will always be with you.

One circle of friends I worked with took this general idea and adapted it. They assigned certain lines to each person present, and then allowed themselves the freedom to improvise, speaking from their hearts.

Sustenance for Heart and Soul

My dear friend Camille, a spiritual counselor who has helped many people heal through illness and live through dying, offered these ideas:

Connect people by having them stand around the bed and hold hands. Send light around the circle, building it in strength, and then, like spokes of a wheel, send that energy into the center, surrounding and supporting the patient.

In certain traditions, people believe the spirit will ideally let go from the feet moving up and out the top of the head. If you visualize the spirit leaving the body, support this movement in helping the spirit to more easily be released from the body. You might want to visualize light moving up through the patient's body, beginning at the feet and passing out through the crown of his or her head.

If appropriate, you can place a hand on the dying person's heart and say, "Whatever pain you may still carry in your heart, release it into my hand."

Visualize the individual's pain being drawn up into the palm of your hand. Then, wave your hand over a candle or through water to purify that pain and release it. Once again, place your hand on the patient's heart, funneling your love through the skin, and fill him or her with love.

These are things that you can do, but you don't need to do anything in particular. My mom simply held her husband of fifty-five years in her arms, surrounding him with her love, and in her heart, allowing him to leave.

Do what feels natural and right in the moment.

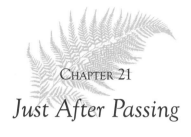

CHAPTER 21

Just After Passing

$\mathcal{W}$hether one has spiritual beliefs or not, we stand in awe at the mystery of life and death. There is a certain need to honor and respect the holiness of this time that feels somehow outside of time. The moments immediately following a death can also be disconcerting. "What are we supposed to do now?"

There truly isn't anything that must be done right away. You can simply sit or stand wherever you are, and breathe slowly. Allow yourself time to absorb some of the enormity of what has happened.

Spontaneous prayer may feel right, silent or spoken. It can be something simple such as: "With love in our hearts, we bless your soul on its way." Or you can just hold the silence for a while if that feels right.

Most of us need a bit of time and space to cushion the shock, and to allow ourselves to simply breathe and be present in the moment. Often, people will cry, hold one another, or kiss and hold the person who has died. After a while, those present may want to share thoughts and feelings.

Practical Matters

While there are some practical things to be attended to, they are not urgent; they can wait for a while. To ease your concerns about

167

what you might need to do, I have addressed the practical steps to consider below:

~ If the patient dies at home and has been under the care of a doctor, there is no need to contact the police, 911, or any other emergency agency.

~ If the patient has been under the care of hospice, but hospice individuals are not present, phone hospice whenever it feels right to do so. If hospice is not involved, you will eventually need to contact the patient's doctor, but you don't need to do so right away.

~ If the patient was not under the care of a doctor or hospice, you will need to contact your local law enforcement agency to request a medical examiner.

~ You will probably want to contact a mortuary, but that does not have to be done until you are ready. Some people feel more comfortable calling the mortuary right away, others prefer to wait several hours before making this call.

Blessing the Spirit

Most religions have prayers that are traditionally offered when a person dies. In some cultures, it is customary to remain at the bedside and continue the vigil for some hours following the death. While honoring the values of the person who has died, be open to what feels right to do or say.

I stayed at the hospital with Tony's body for almost three hours after he died, until an inner voice told me that it was time to leave. Intuition guided me throughout Tony's last few days, and in the time that followed his passing. Immediately after his death, an inner sense prompted me to spontaneously bless his spirit. I have no idea whether I spoke aloud, but my gratitude, my love, my respect and admiration for Tony flowed from me like a river into the current that had lifted his spirit.

If your loved one was connected with a faith tradition, you might want to draw upon the prayers and rites of that religion. For those with no specific spiritual affiliation, the following serves as an example.

Henry's family gathered in a circle around his bed shortly after he died. One family member invited the others in the room to place their hands on Henry if that felt comfortable. Closing their eyes and breathing deeply, they held one another and Henry in a sphere of light.

Henry, you journey now beyond our world.
May your soul be blessed by having known and loved us,
as we have been blessed by loving and knowing you.

Those present then expressed their individual thoughts about Henry. Then, the family said the following blessing to close the ritual.

May the love travel with you, Henry.
May all love surround you.
May the divine source of love guide you
as your soul journeys on from here.

You could also include a prayer with this blessing, if that's appropriate. Honor the values of the deceased, and honor your own needs, too. It is important not to feel rushed after someone you love dies. It is okay for those present to spend a long time just being, thinking, remembering, crying, praying, and talking to the person who has died.

Some people are not comfortable remaining in the room, that's okay, too. Others may want to have time alone in the room with the deceased. Honor your own needs, and be respectful of others' needs.

In many traditions, people believe the spirit lingers near the body for some time after the death. Whether this is your belief or not, it is appropriate to be respectful of the possibility and behave as if your loved one is aware of all that is said or done.

If you are somewhere other than in a hospital room, you may choose to light candles at this time. If there has been oxygen for the patient, be sure to not only turn it off, but remove it from the room—small amounts of oxygen could be leaking from the tank and you don't want an added tragedy.

Gathering to Say Farewell

Close friends and family can be contacted and given the opportunity to come and be present if they want. There is as much time as you need for this. It often feels more intimate to say goodbye at home, or even in a hospital room, than during the more formal situation at the mortuary.

If there will be direct cremation, this will be the last time to be with this person. Take the time you need.

There are people who would not be comfortable with any humor at such a time, but for others, humor is not at all inappropriate.

When I arrived at the hospital shortly after my father's death, I hugged my mother and we cried. As we waited for the others in the family to get there, Mom often leaned over and kissed Daddy, holding his face in her hands. Then she would stand and talk with me. A comment overheard from a nurse in the hallway reminded Mom of a funny story about Daddy, and before long, we found ourselves giggling. For a moment, I was horrified, my father's body wasn't cold yet and here we were laughing! But it also felt absolutely right that we were crying and laughing together.

As my brothers and their adult children entered the hospital room, we hugged one another and cried. But after a while, we were all laughing. We wondered if others might think this meant we didn't care. We knew, though, that all of us, and Daddy too, understood that being able to laugh was as honest, healthy, and as loving as the tears we shed.

Some people are compelled to touch the person who has died, while others are not at all comfortable with doing so. Whatever the inclination, it is right, and should be honored.

A little while after my Uncle Ray's death, his sister began phoning people from her church. I needed quiet space to reflect, so I took a walk around the neighborhood. Honor your own needs while being respectful of the needs of others.

Once people have all gathered together, the family might want to do a blessing. (If someone isn't comfortable participating, allow him or her to step away from the room.) Prayer from the heart, or prayer from tradition is appropriate, as is the blessing earlier in this chapter.

The following prayer was created to reflect Jesse's beliefs, and to allow Jesse's family to express their love for him.

May Jesse be conscious of our love, we of his.

May the love illuminating all of our beings shine through each one of us and into the soul of Jesse as he moves away from earthly life.

Let our gratitude shine upon him, filling him with the sweetness of earthly love.

Let the radiance of infinity shine upon him, filling him with the light of divine love.

Washing the Body

This is an age-old custom that only in the past century has been handed off to professionals. Most definitely not for everyone, but it is an option that can be very healing and meaningful for some.

(Please note that in a situation where there might be any question regarding the cause of death, it is best not to wash the body. In certain cases, it might even be considered tampering with evidence.)

A ritual washing of the beloved's body is a rite of purification, and an offering of human or exalted blessing. Participating in the ritual demonstrates a reverence for the sacred vessel that housed the human spirit of the beloved.

If you have already learned how to bathe a bedfast patient, then you know the technique. If not, you can ask hospice to demonstrate. You could keep it simple and wash only the front of the body, or the face and hands. All you need is a washcloth, a large bowl of warm soapy water, and a basin of clear water.

In many traditions, washing the body is accompanied by prayer. You could light candles, and scent the water with lavender or rosemary. Perhaps you will want to bless the parts of the body as they are bathed.

"We are so grateful to have seen love shining through these eyes, and we are grateful that these eyes saw such beauty in this world.

"We bless these shoulders that bore the weight of (list burdens or duties).

"We bless these hands that baked bread, held babies, crafted furniture, (whatever the person did with his or her hands)."

"We bless this heart that loved ...

"We bless this stomach that digested food and brought nourishment to her body.

"We bless these legs that skipped rope when she was young, ran on the track team in high school, as a mom chased after her children, walked beside friends and family offering support..."

Allow yourself the freedom to recall whatever holds meaning in the moment. This is a last opportunity to physically connect with your loved one's body. If you are drawn to this ritual, allow your instincts to guide you through it with love.

Simply washing your loved one's face and hands with reverence can serve as a symbolic washing of the body, and this is something more people might be comfortable doing.

While I had thought that I would want to wash Tony's body when the time came, the thought didn't even occur to me in the hours after his passing. Instinctively though, I picked up a washcloth and washed his face three times, then washed his hands as had become our nightly ritual.

An alternate rite of purification is smudging, which means to wave smoking sage or incense over and around the person, room, or object that is being blessed and purified. If you are in a location where this would be permissible, smudge the body as you lovingly release the spirit.

Blessings to Release the Body

Many prayers in this book can be said before death, immediately after, or before relinquishing the body to hospital or mortuary staff. You might use different prayers at different times, or repeat the same one with needed changes to the wording. The words really are not as important as creating a space for those present to offer love and say their goodbyes.

> [Name] we love you.
> We will miss you so much.
> You will always be with us in our hearts.
> We bless you for having been,
> and we bless you on your way.

Each person may offer a personal goodbye, and then pause for a moment of silence.

Silent prayer works well when different spiritual points of view must be considered. A blessing can also provide a setting for honoring different beliefs, such as a Baptist prayer said for the parents followed by a Buddhist chant for the daughter.

Participating in ritual following a death helps us feel more connected to what has happened, and more connected to one another—particularly important at this time because we often are feeling rather disconnected. It is helpful to include an affirmation of the connection between those still living, as well as the connection between those living and dead. This could be done by first holding the deceased in the light, and then holding one another in the light.

The following are two additional blessings that could be used together or separately:

Closing our eyes and joining together in a spirit of prayer, let us become aware of the divine source of love, which surrounds and suffuses us all.

Let us allow the warm glow of this spirit to be felt in each of our hearts.

May this divine source of love, the source of all life, grace us with a heightened sense of the power and mystery of life; and of love, extending beyond all boundaries.

Spirit of divine wisdom and infinite love, welcome [name], and sustain her/his spirit in the joyful radiance of eternity.

Connections of the heart transcend all boundaries.

We will always be connected to [name].

These heart connections also

connect all of us in our sorrow,

though we each may express it in our own way.

May we be brave and kind enough to honor the differences as we support one another in the time of grief that lies ahead.

Meaningful Mementos

Some people are comforted by cutting a lock of hair as a gesture of remembrance. Some may choose to remove a wedding ring or other meaningful piece of jewelry. Many men and women wear a partner's wedding ring, sometimes on a chain around the neck. Those in grief often find comfort through symbols that affirm, "Something of you will always be with me." A memento provides a tangible expression that the bond is still felt. People die, but love does not.

Some might want to place an item of special significance on or near the loved one's body, such as a rosary, favorite photo, or other symbol of connection with a beloved. These symbolic activities can resonate in hearts and minds for years in a way that goes beyond logical understanding. If cremation will take place, it may make sense to remove these items before that occurs. After cremation, you can place the mementos in the urn if that seems appropriate.

When the hospital staff or mortuary personnel arrive to take the body, it is usually best to leave the room, though I do know of occasions where the professionals were exceptionally sensitive to family members' special wishes. One son wanted to help transfer his father's body to the mortuary vehicle parked out front. Another family took comfort in grooming the elderly woman, and their young daughter entered into the process by suggesting that Grandma would like her special blanket and a favorite book.

Many people, though, find that taking a walk at this time feels more comfortable, and the fresh air is welcome after having been inside for some time. It is often both shocking, and grounding, that the world outside is still going about its business despite the enormity of what you have just experienced. Trucks rumble down the street, people walk their dogs, and birds chirp and soar overhead. Inconceivable as it may seem, life does go on.

CHAPTER 22

The Days Between Death
and the Funeral or Memorial

$\mathcal{I}$n the first day or two following the death of a loved one, there are a number of matters that must be attended to, such as contacting family, friends, and colleagues, making funeral arrangements, writing an obituary, and trying to sort through so many unexpected feelings. It is all overwhelming.

Even when a death is expected, we are dazed, in shock and grief, and yet, somehow we make our way through as best as we can. We don't all respond to loss in the same way. Some people throw themselves into the tasks. Some may barely be able to form a coherent thought. Others vacillate between these two extremes. Regardless of your response, you will need support and a sense of connection. People usually want to help but often don't know exactly how. If there are things that others can do to help you, ask for their assistance.

Participation in one or more of the rituals in this chapter can help you be a little more grounded in this new reality that seems unreal. These rituals can strengthen connections with others, offer ways to do something for the deceased, and provide a means to learn how to have an ongoing relationship with the loved one now gone.

Remembering Together

Periodically, we hear that an event will be held to commemorate a person or occasion. Commemorate means "to remember together." When family and friends come together and share their memories with one another, even in a casual setting, they are commemorating the individual. In the fragile days after the death of a loved one, it is comforting to share stories about the person.

In most circumstances, it is healing to share not just the person's virtues but also frustrations with his or her irritating habits. I encourage you to commemorate the heroics and humor, foibles and fears, wit and wisdom, warmth and weaknesses—the full kaleidoscope of the personality.

Generally, sharing stories happens spontaneously, but some interesting questions to ask yourself and others are:

Of all the memory movies running through your head, if you had to pick one image to keep, what would it be?

What was the greatest impact he or she had on you, and on your life?

What were a couple of small, but important ways this person influenced you?

What used to drive you crazy about this person?

Many people discover that talking about the deceased with others brings a powerful sense of connection. As one woman expressed it, "Talking about my brother helped me connect with the spirit of his truly unique personality. It also made me realize he will live on, not only in the hearts of those who deeply love him, but also in the lives of all those who made the effort to understand him. Sharing stories about my brother with family and close friends brought us into connection with one another, too, which helped us feel a little less lonely."

In some circles and cultures, one does not speak ill of the dead. In recent decades in Western culture, though, there has been a move toward greater honesty. While it is inappropriate to make accusations that the individual cannot now refute, honesty graced with affection is a healthier approach to remembrance. It isn't necessary to make the one who has died more admirable or better than he or she was in order to show respect or love. When we acknowledge all of who the person was, and hold him or her in our love, then we are loving the fullness of the individual rather than a constrained or distorted image. Doing so in a communal setting is healing.

At a memorial gathering for my friend Doug, one man spoke of Doug's sterling qualities and then also mentioned Doug's overly precise nature. With gentle humor, the friend told of his occasional frustration with Doug in this regard. Everyone in attendance felt affection for Doug, but they were also well aware of his tendency to be overly precise. It was part of what defined Doug, and since he was held in high regard, it became affectionate to recall this irritating side of him. Furthermore, I think it helped to lessen everyone's guilt around their occasional impatience with Doug when he went too far.

Understanding this as a natural human response, we can forgive ourselves for not always being infinitely understanding. We can love others in the totality of their fullness and their awkwardness as human beings.

Another way of sharing memories is to make a collage of the person's life to display at the visitation and memorial or funeral service. It could be two-dimensional with photos, poems, or paintings. The display could also be three-dimensional with pottery, musical instruments, handmade quilts, woodwork, or whatever is representative of the individual. Afterward, the collage can be displayed at home or at work.

Adding Personal Touches to the Funeral

Through sharing memories, the family can gain a sense of what to memorialize at the funeral, as well as what is appropriate in terms of style. A traditional setting and format are well suited to many people, but that is not the only way to go.

Funeral and memorial services can take place at home, in gardens, even public parks with permission. Sometimes, a more unusual setting is appropriate, such as an art gallery, historic location, or ball field. Nontraditional aspects might be fitting to include, depending on the individual you are commemorating.

Henry, an avid bird watcher, said often during his illness that he wasn't afraid to die, he knew his spirit would be able to fly with the birds. The day following his death there seemed to be more birds than usual around the house, and Henry's daughter commented, "Wouldn't it be lovely if all these birds also attended my father's funeral."

A family friend had recently attended a wedding that included a dove release. As a special tribute to Henry, the friend arranged to have a dove release at the conclusion of the cemetery service.

Whether you have a funeral, memorial service, or a celebration of life, being involved with the planning provides a way to do one last thing for the deceased. Deciding upon photos, music, and poetry, as well as personal stories to be integrated into the service, can be a helpful and healing process.

Chapter 28 includes an overview of a funeral service, along with three sample ceremonies for those who want to create a more personalized ceremony for their loved one.

Holding a Place for Love

Grief is not an ordinary state of mind, and often, people feel a need for things that seem unusual. Be open and accepting of the fact that we are all different and we all grieve differently. What provides comfort to one person might be discomforting to another.

For instance, a mother may be adamant about keeping a child's room intact and visit the room nightly at tuck-in time to commune with her child. All of the love still exists, and the desire to take care of her child finds expression through this ritual. Another parent might avoid even entering the room until quite some time has passed.

I know many widows and widowers who love that a favorite shirt or sweater still smells like their spouse, and they refuse to wash it. Children, both young and grown, may also feel similarly about a deceased parent's favorite article of clothing. They may even wrap themselves in a familiar jacket or bathrobe for comfort during times of grief.

Previously insignificant items can take on symbolic meaning after a death. Conscious and unconscious rituals may develop that offer support, sustenance, and a sense of connection. Even if it might seem strange to others, hold on to what comforts you and honor what will help you heal.

In some cultures, the family continues to set a place at the table for the deceased for a few days to several weeks following the death. This is considered an act of respect and devotion. People believe that if the spirit of the deceased visits the home, the spirit will know he or she is remembered, and continues to be cared for. Some believe the spirit actually partakes of the essence of the food, even though the material food remains.

At first glance, this seems an unlikely ritual in contemporary Western culture, yet it offers something to those who mourn a loss.

I know of contemporary widows who have found this practice to be greatly comforting. One woman, Therese, felt that if her husband's spirit could see the material world, he would be touched by what she was doing and this would nourish his soul. Every night for the first week after his death, Therese set a place for her husband at the dinner table. She continued the ritual once a week for three months. After that, Therese did so on the monthly date of his death until the first anniversary of his passing. After that, she felt it was time for him, and for her, to move on with acceptance that they would be separated until she joined him. Therese said this ritual provided a way to demonstrate that this man she loved so much still had a place in her life.

Another widow, Gina, practiced a similar ritual after the death of her husband. Gina and her young daughter created special evenings they called "Daddy Night." Both were free to talk to him and tell him whatever they wanted, and they included him in their general table discussions on those nights. Sometimes, one would say to the other, "I think Daddy would say this about that." Over time, it became less sorrowful and more fun for them. After awhile, they phased out the ritual, but occasionally, one or the other would express a desire for a Daddy Night, and the ritual was there waiting for them.

Another woman, Sophie, did a simpler ritual to honor her husband. In the morning, she placed his coffee cup on the breakfast table in his usual spot. Sophie explained, "It just makes me feel better seeing it there."

Sophie admitted she was slightly embarrassed to tell me about this because she thought it was a bit odd. I assured her there was nothing wrong with developing personal rituals that offer comfort.

When mourning a loss, it is helpful to participate in activities and rituals that heal and support you as you hold a place for the beloved in your heart and in your life.

PART FOUR

Specific Circumstances

CHAPTER 23

General Guidelines for Children

*I*t's important to remember that children are people, whether they are a patient, family member, or visitor. Children have fears, and wants, and difficulty with change—just like grownups. They also have questions, and concerns. They sometimes feel guilty that something they said or did may have caused the illness, and need to be reassured they are not at fault.

Levels of comprehension will vary from one age to another, and according to each child's unique personality. No matter how young, though, children want to be treated with respect, and prefer it if we are honest with them. They sense when something is wrong, and if we are not honest with them, it interferes with trust and can make the child more anxious. Shielding children from realities is not as effective as supporting them in age appropriate ways.

Children have different needs at different stages of development, and how we interact with a child of three is different than how we would explain something to a child of seven, or twelve years of age. The website, hospicenet.org provides guidelines for the particular needs of different age groups. (The homepage includes a section on children, which includes "Talking to Children About Death" and "Children's Understanding of Death," both of which offer helpful advice.) Hospital social workers may also be able to help, and a local hospice agency may be able to offer suggestions even if the patient is not participating in hospice. Below are some general points to keep in mind, whether the child is the patient or a family member.

Answer questions honestly.

Keep the information simple and age appropriate.

Invite the child to ask questions and express feelings.

Expressing your thoughts and feelings in a simple way can help the child understand why others are behaving differently than usual.

Some examples:

~ [Mommy, Rebecca, Grandma] is sick and we're concerned. The doctors are trying to figure out what is wrong, and how they might fix it.

~ She has a very bad sickness, it's called _____. The doctors may not be able to help her get well, but I'm hoping something can be done.

~ The doctors have tried everything they know to help her, but she isn't getting better. This makes me and your aunts and uncles feel very sad.

Even if the patient has an encouraging prognosis, children may still have questions about death and dying. Don't brush them aside, honor their questions with thoughtful answers.

Respect the child's timing. He or she may not be ready to talk when you are. Provide openings, and be patient. Expect that the thoughts and feelings will come out a little at a time. If you listen carefully, take what is said seriously, and answer questions honestly, the child will become more open about expressing thoughts and feelings that may be difficult to put into words.

Invite questions, and answer each question simply and honestly. Some children will ask many questions, while others may be satisfied with a single, brief response. Often, a child will revisit the issue a few days later with an additional question or two, such as: What happens then? Will she die? What does that mean?

These questions can be difficult for parents to answer, but the response can be fairly simple. One way to answer a child's question of "What happens when people die?" is to explain it in terms the child can understand. As an example: "Remember when the batteries wore out on your toy, and it wouldn't move or make noise? People don't have batteries like toys, but sometimes when people are very sick or very old, something wears out. After someone dies, the body can't see or hear or move. The body doesn't breathe and doesn't feel pain, it doesn't feel anything. Unlike your toy, though, we can't just get new batteries to fix it. There isn't anything we can do to fix it, no matter how much we want to."

It is not unusual for children to regress or act out during stressful times. Expecting this to happen on occasion can help in understanding that insecurity is what underlies the behavior. While it is good to be flexible, there should still be some boundaries that are gently and consistently enforced. Clear boundaries can help a child feel more secure, and provide a sense of normalcy.

Explaining Death

The child may ask, "What happens to us after we die?"

You might respond, "Nobody knows for sure, but many people believe that we go to a much nicer place." Then explain your own beliefs in simple terms. It may be helpful to also explain other points of view if they are part of the common culture of the child.

While using metaphors can be helpful, be careful about euphemisms, such as "Grandpa has just gone to sleep." Young children tend to take things quite literally and this can cause a child to be afraid of going to sleep for fear they won't ever wake up. Using the phrase "going away on a long trip" can cause a child great distress when later told Mommy or Daddy is going on a trip.

Explaining death can be difficult. Reading an age-appropriate book with the child can ease the process and open the door for questions. If you don't have time to find the right book, enlist the help of someone who knows the child. A short list of books is included in Resources.

If the Child Is the Patient

While the majority of the rituals in this book are adult oriented, many of them could be shaped for a child who is ill. Children and teens often have a strong sense of what they need, and if given a little encouragement many will offer their own ideas of what they want to do.

There is a desire to protect children, but be careful not to overprotect them. Allowing the child a sense of autonomy, and age-appropriate independence is a powerful way of supporting the child's emotional and mental health.

When possible, offer choices so that he or she will have a sense of some control over their life. Some examples:

Would you prefer your appointment scheduled for the morning or the afternoon?

Which arm for your blood draw?

Would you like me to see if I can stay overnight with you in the hospital?

Be cautious about indulging every whim. Even if the child protests or complains, adhering to established guidelines provides a sense of normalcy and is comforting.

Maintain clear boundaries with regard to demanding, selfish, or other inappropriate behaviors. Not feeling well can make people irritable, and we need to be patient with them, but no one is served by being allowed to behave like a tyrant.

Hospital staff can help parents understand the special needs of seriously ill children—not only medical needs, but also the social and psychological needs. If no one offers you this kind of support, ask a nurse, the hospitalist, or a social worker for suggestions as to how you can better understand not only your ill child, but also the needs of other children in the family.

If special programs or hand-outs are available, take advantage of them.

If the Child's Family Member Is the Patient

Because so much time and energy is focused on the patient, the healthy child may feel as if he or she is less important. Create special time to spend with this child, who may feel left out. Children need to know that their thoughts, feelings, and fears matter to you.

Ask friends or family to help provide support by spending special time with the well child.

Identify occasions when family or friends can provide a helping hand that will allow Mom or Dad to spend extra time with the well child.

A child will be more willing to accept the circumstance if parents practice honesty, consideration, and allow him or her to make choices where possible. Because the well child may be expected to take on a bit more responsibility, it is only fair to allow him or her a little more autonomy.

If the Child Is a Visitor to the Patient

The involvement of children who are connected to the patient can be helpful and meaningful, but there are a few guidelines:

Let the child know what to expect, then let the child choose whether or not to be involved.

Provide an "out" for the child should there be a change of mind.

During critical periods and at the funeral, it is extremely helpful to have an adult not grieving who is able to focus on the needs of the child.

Chapter 24

Alzheimer's and Dementia Patients

*R*ituals are generally no different for Alzheimer's and other dementia patients in terms of intent. However, the context is sometimes not the same, and certain adjustments may need to be made for these patients just as with other activities.

The timing of what needs to be addressed becomes more critical in some areas, and more fluid in others. For example, it would be important to address paperwork, medical directives, and resolution of difficult relationships as early as possible. Caring for patients with dementia is often draining, but listed below are some suggestions to invite meaningful connections through the different stages.

Mild Dementia

Spending time in nature is nourishing for most people, but can be particularly important for Alzheimer's patients because physical exercise and sensory stimulation can help slow the decline.

Alzheimer's and dementia patients may not be able to enter into life review in the same way that others might, but there are times when family and friends can help these patients flesh out what they do remember. Ask questions, and enquire about details such as setting, time of year, or who was present. Ask how he or she felt at the time. The emotional or sensory aspects may help these patients to connect to other memories. You can ask, "Were there other times in your life when ... ?" Old photos can sometimes spark memories. And be sure to remind your loved one of their achievements.

When trying to provoke reminiscences, be careful to avoid saying, "Don't you remember...?" This can cause patients to feel uncomfortable they don't remember, and may prompt them to pretend they do. Be especially careful with this in regard to recent events.

Shared activities such as gardening, crafts, art projects, or hobbies, are ways to spend meaningful time together. This can be beneficial for caregiver as well as patient. Creating a ritual aspect to begin the activity, such as always saying the same thing as you clear the table and bring out the box of supplies, provides a sense of familiarity and can help the patient anticipate what is coming. This repetition of behavior helps some Alzheimer's and dementia patients feel more comfortable entering into an activity.

Turning patient care into caring rituals (see Chapter 18) supports caregivers as much as patients. Other rituals in the same chapter, such as enhancing environment, might be employed even though the patient is still in good physical health.

Alzheimer's and dementia patients can easily become agitated, frustrated, irritable, and sometimes quite aggressive. For some unknown reason, many of these patients are calmed by ice cream. You might create a pleasant ritual with this cold treat to avert difficult behavior.

Naomi's dad often became irritable in the late afternoon. At the first hint of this, Naomi would suggest that they take an ice cream break. She put aside her work and they would sit at the kitchen table and have a small dish of ice cream together. Naomi kept the conversation lighthearted and used it as a break from her chores, a short respite to relax and enjoy a pleasant interlude with her father.

Saying, "I'm sorry—I love you—Thank you," should be said before the patient loses any more of their memory, but these things can certainly be said even after the patient has difficulty comprehending. The patient's heart will understand the feelings expressed.

Moderate Stage

When patients are not here in this "now," the options for connecting become more limited, but you can open to new possibilities. Be willing to meet him wherever he is and connect with him there. If Dad is living in 1946, let go of today and visit 1946 with him. More than just accepting that this is where he is right now, honor that this is where he is by entering into that time and place with him.

Many tribal cultures believe that in powerful ritual, time becomes flexible. You can borrow this concept and enter into ritual time, letting go for a while of the constraints of "here and now." Thus freed, allow yourself to be childlike and let go of your rational mind. Embark upon a treasure hunt to discover what joy or solace you can bring to the patient in whatever world he or she inhabits in that moment.

Songs, particularly from youth, are an excellent method of connection for dementia patients. It seems that music is stored in the brain in a different way than other information, and so is somehow more accessible. According to studies, providing music therapy to Alzheimer's patients reduces agitation and aggression, stimulates memory, and provides a form of social interaction.

Spend thirty minutes a day playing music the Alzheimer's patient enjoys. This is even better if you also engage with the music by singing along, asking questions, or commenting. Many senior centers provide musical activities and attending these can provide patients with a social context for experiencing live music.

When an Alzheimer's patient doesn't know you, or thinks you are someone else, it can be painful to experience. Instead of fighting it—a useless battle—try your best to go with it. Accept that you are someone "new" or different to this person now.

George remembered his young wife, Alene, very well, but did not connect her with the woman who currently shared his bed. It was sad and difficult for Alene that her husband no longer knew who she was, but sweet that he was still so in love with the young woman he married. Together, they explored his memories of Alene—even though George didn't know the person he was sharing them with was, in fact, Alene. A less than perfect situation, but it was a way for Alene to connect with her husband, and their treasured past.

Explore how you can connect with your loved one without an established history. My aunt suffered from dementia and did not know my name or any details of our shared history, but there was still an emotional connection between us and I valued that. Though feeling the loss acutely, still we create bridges to connect.

Severe Dementia

When the patient's communication deteriorates to the point where few if any words are spoken, the avenues to connect become fewer. You can still express your own thoughts and explore memories in the patient's presence, though you likely won't receive a coherent response. Trust, though, that what you say is heard, and felt—and even understood—on some level. Just as with any patient who no longer seems fully present, the connection of the heart is strong and if you bring your love into the room, the patient will feel it.

Even if the patient isn't bedfast, some of the rituals in Chapter 19 can be useful in creating bridges to connect. Also, rituals such as co-meditation, and offering a litany of gratitude and love can be helpful at this stage.

If you think there are things the patient would like to be able to say to you, say it for them—especially "Thank you," "I love you," or "I'm sorry." As an example: "Mom, I know that you loved me—even during those years when we were often at odds with one another. I know you did the best you could. Somewhere inside, I even knew it then. I'll forgive you for not always being a perfect mother, if you'll forgive me for not always being a perfect daughter. I know you love me, and I hope you knew how much I loved you then, and how much I love you still."

Throughout the progression of this dreadful disease, family and friends must continually adjust to the patient's changing abilities and needs, and develop new ways to connect. It is helpful to utilize "both-and" thinking in a number of areas. Aspects of the patient's personality are no longer present, so it can feel as if he or she is gone, but isn't really gone. This difficult ambiguity becomes more tolerable when using both-and to frame the situation. "My dad is not fully present, and he is still here." You also need to honor both the patient's needs, and your own. You *both* love the person, and are frustrated by some of the behavior. It is a balancing act. Remembering to employ both-and thinking can help you find needed perspective.

Pauline Boss, Ph.D., author of *Loving Someone Who Has Dementia: How to Find Hope While Coping with Stress and Grief*, writes with eloquence and understanding about such losses. She provides insight into the particular difficulties families of dementia patients face daily. In an earlier book, *Ambiguous Loss: Learning to Live with*

Unresolved Grief, she observes, "...existing rituals and community supports only address clear-cut loss."

You can create your own rituals, though. Find objects to symbolize what is gone, and just as would be done at a funeral, acknowledge the loss. Allow yourself time to grieve, and then affirm the joy in having experienced these blessings. You might want to wrap these symbols in velvet and place them in a special box. Then find objects to symbolize what is not lost, and place these on an altar of gratitude as a reminder of what you still have.

You might find it helpful to write about what is lost. This will help you to express your feelings of grief. The words written on paper will serve as tangible evidence that those memories are still strong and vivid, and are not truly lost.

I encourage you to take advantage of the many resources for support, a number of which are listed in "Resources." Most communities offer at least a few programs that can help patients and their caregivers. It is worth the time it takes to seek out the variety of help available, including day care, activities, support groups, information, and workshops. Greater understanding not only lifts the weight of the caregiver's burdens, but can also bring more meaningful interaction into the relationship with a dementia patient.

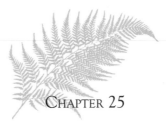

CHAPTER 25

Unexpected Sudden Death

*B*ill's health had been steadily deteriorating, multiple diseases taking their toll. Hospice staff were visiting a few times a week, and Bill's wife, Stacy, was expecting that any time they would tell her he was in his last week of life. However, Bill stabilized.

One evening while Stacy and Bill were watching television together, he suddenly went into cardiac arrest. Stacy called 911. When the paramedics arrived, they tried to revive him, but were unsuccessful. They put Bill into an ambulance, and transported him to the hospital emergency room. Efforts there were also futile.

Stacy was in shock. She had thought her husband would have a peaceful death at home. Instead, Bill's last moments had been chaotic, with no time for the loving rituals she had hoped to provide in his last days and hours. Stacy telephoned me from the hospital. Between sobs she told me, "It's like when I went to all of the natural childbirth classes, and then had to have an emergency C-section. Except this is worse—so, so much worse."

I suggested she tell the nurse that she wanted to spend time with Bill, and if she had difficulty to ask for the hospital chaplain or social worker. "You can still surround Bill with your love. In many cultures, it is believed that the spirit remains near the body for some time after death. You can offer Bill a last litany of gratitude."

I drove to the hospital and Stacy and I phoned close family members, some of whom expressed a desire to come to the hospital. When they arrived we offered a prayer together, blessed Bill's spirit, and there was an opportunity for everyone to spend time with Bill and say goodbye.

Many of the rituals in Chapters 19, 20 and 21 are an option with sudden death, though certain adjustments might need to be made. You may want to offer a litany of gratitude and love, bless his or her spirit, and say goodbye. If the patient was taken to an emergency room, hospital staff can usually provide you and your loved one with a more private room.

Hospital chaplains are a good source for help with practical details, as well as offering spiritual and emotional support. Chaplains are trained to respect all spiritual points of view, including atheist. He or she should honor your faith perspective, so don't be shy about telling the chaplain what you want.

Chapter 26

Removing Artificial Life Support

Choosing to remove life support for someone you love is painful and difficult, wrought with conflicting feelings. The strides of medicine have put patients' families in situations that wouldn't have been possible twenty-five years ago. How do we move through such a circumstance? The same way we move through the other parts of life—not one hundred percent sure, but doing the best we know how.

Points to Consider

The key question to ask when grappling with the decision is, "Are we truly extending life, or are we prolonging the dying process?" And even more important, "What would the patient want?"

It is common for those close to the patient to feel:

"There might be a chance she could pull through."

"I can't just let him die if there is anything else that could possibly be done."

"Please, do anything and everything you can because I don't want to be without this person I love."

None of us wants to lose a loved one, but none of us wants our loved ones to suffer unnecessarily either. Is it likely that the patient's life can be saved, or is their suffering and discomfort being stretched out over a longer period of time than is warranted?

~ Request a sit-down, family meeting with doctors, nurses, hospital chaplains, and social workers, to gain the best understanding of the medical and ethical realities of your particular situation. The professionals involved may not all have the same opinion, and this can be confusing and unsettling. Part of what makes artificial life support such a difficult issue for professionals, as well as family members, is that there is a large area of gray in between the black and white.

If the patient has not stated preferences verbally or in a medical directive, do your best to intuit what the patient would want under the circumstances. If you do not already have a palliative care team, ask to meet with this team of professional caregivers. They can help you clarify goals of care, assist with the decision making process, and insure that the patient has full comfort care whichever choice you make. This team also provides emotional and practical support for the patients' family members.

~ A key fact to understand: By removing a feeding tube, you are not starving a patient to death, you are allowing the body to die naturally. Allowing nature to take its course is not the same as hastening death. As part of the gradual shutting down process, the body stops taking in food. Feeding tubes are an artificial support and can cause physical discomfort to the patient. Quality of life must be considered. Ask yourself, "What would the patient want?"

~ Check with medical personnel for a general idea of what to expect after the artificial support has been suspended. Death is not usually instantaneous. The time could vary from a few hours to a few days, possibly even a week or more.

Interacting with a Patient Through Ritual

Though generally the patient will not be conscious, it is nonetheless a matter of respect to tell the person what you are going to do and why. It is possible that some remote consciousness, or spirit, will understand and appreciate this consideration.

Let the patient know when life support will be removed and how. If there is a nurse, doctor, or clergyperson with whom the patient or family has a strong connection, having him or her present might help you feel more comfortable.

You might do a prayer or ritual such as might be done in the final days. See Chapters 19 and 20. Also, offer the patient your gratitude and love.

Some people find it comforting to bring special items into the room—items relating to the patient's career or hobby, a favorite piece of clothing, or objects that hold meaning. The significance will vary from one situation to another, but these items can help to personalize the hospital setting and ease the goodbye process.

The following are four examples of what you might want to say.

Because your body cannot function without extreme measures, and because it does not seem possible that you could get better, we have decided to remove artificial life support to your body. In about an hour the nurse will come and begin to disconnect the machines.

> We feel certain that you wouldn't want to live a life without more quality than this. Your family is here with you [list names]. We are in agreement on this, but filled with sorrow. We will miss you. You have added so very much to our lives. Our love and appreciation for you will not end when you leave us.

Allow each person time to be with the patient, perhaps alone, and to say whatever needs to be said.

Before the removal of life support, form a circle around the patient, and hold him or her in the light of your love.

Generally, family members leave the room as tubes are removed. After the equipment has been taken away, you may want to return to the patient's bedside for another circle of support to reinforce that the patient is still held in your love. Sometimes this helps family members affirm that the patient is not being abandoned.

> (This can be done with or without the references to God.)
> Because your soul is no longer able to express itself here,
> but not able to leave and soar [toward God]
> we choose to release that part of you that can soar,
> freeing it from the body which no longer can.
>
> Rather than interfering any further, we choose to allow
> the processes of [God and] nature to take their course.
> Should [God and] nature conspire to return you to yourself,
> and thereby return you to us, we would be overjoyed.

If it is right for you to move away from us,
we will no longer hold you here,
but will allow your spirit to be set free.

(The second version of the following example does not include the references to God.)

Dear God, creator of this wondrous universe, which is so much more than we can possibly comprehend, we are doing our best to trust in your greater wisdom and infinite love.

Help us to feel your guidance and comforting support as we move through these difficult days.

We offer our thanks for the bounty of gifts you have provided us throughout our lives, including the blessing of sharing part of our lives with [name].

We come to you today with heavy hearts, asking that you hold [name] in your loving embrace.

We understand that his mortal mind no longer fully comprehends, but we ask that the consciousness of his spirit will feel you surrounding and supporting him with your divine love.

We ask also that his spirit be aware of the earthly love that radiates from those who gather at his bedside—[perhaps mention names of those present]—all who come to offer their love and say goodbye.

It is with great sadness that life support will be withdrawn, but the decision is prompted by a greater love that knows [name] would rather be set free than stay trapped too long in a body unable to respond to life and those he loves.

In humbled sadness, we ask for your love and support for all of us. Amen.

Version without References to God:

This wondrous universe is so much more than we can possibly comprehend.

We are doing our best to trust in a greater wisdom and an infinite love.

May we all feel guidance and comforting support as we move through these difficult days.

We feel gratitude for the bounty of gifts received throughout our lives, including the blessing of sharing part of our lives with [name].

We come here today with heavy hearts, to hold [name] in our loving embrace.

We understand that his mortal mind no longer fully comprehends, but we ask that the consciousness of his spirit will feel us surrounding and supporting him with our love.

It is with great sadness that life support will be withdrawn, but the decision is prompted by a greater love that knows [name] would rather be set free than stay trapped too long in a body unable to respond to life and those he loves.

In humbled sadness, we offer our love and support to [name], and to one another.

This one could be used following a prayer from the patient's chosen faith.

> During the time in which [name] remains with us, dear Lord, help her spirit to be aware of the love expressed by those who come alone or with others to say goodbye, and to share with her the ways in which they are better for having her in their life.
>
> May some part of her rejoice in hearing the ways in which she will live on in our hearts, and as an influence in our lives. May we all feel free to share favorite memories with her as we offer our love and gratitude to bless her on her way into your welcoming heart.
>
> [Use the appropriate closing of the patient's faith, such as, "In Jesus' name we ask this, amen."]

After life support is removed, you might use prayer to direct the soul toward God, or to declare your love and your loved one's value.

CHAPTER 27

Home-Centered After-Death Care

For many centuries, it was customary when someone died for the body to be "laid out" in the home until the funeral. Often, the family participated in preparing the body. While this might seem a little unusual to contemporary Americans, a number of cultures keep the body at home for twenty-four hours or more as a sign of love and respect. There has been a small but growing movement to reclaim this tradition.

Although home-centered after-death care is an option that few would be comfortable doing, I know of a number of situations where this was exactly right and deeply meaningful. Several of these situations involved a circle of friends who researched the practical and legal aspects of home-centered care of the deceased. They then did everything themselves, even preparing the body and handcrafting the casket. (Information on detailed guidance can be found in "Resources.")

I know of several other cases where the family employed the help of a funeral director rather than taking on the full responsibility, yet were more involved than is the usual practice in our culture. Karen and her husband, David, made the experience into just what they needed when their nine-year-old daughter, Sally, died. Karen remembered her grandmother telling her about relatives being "laid out" at home until the funeral, and Karen wanted to have Sally with her at home for a few more days. The funeral director prepared her daughter's body, and then brought her back home in a casket.

Meanwhile, Karen cleaned Sally's bedroom and brought out special things of hers to place around the young girl's room where the body would be laid out. For this grieving mother, it was an act of love to set up the girl's bedroom with flowers, photographs, special toys, and other meaningful items.

Instead of only two hours for visitation at the mortuary, the parents welcomed into their home the warmth and support of neighbors, friends, and extended family during designated times over a two-day period.

Karen and David slept in Sally's room, and felt that spending extra time with Sally's body made it easier to let her go.

David said it gave them some sense of control at a time when everything felt so out of control. He liked that the visitation period could happen on the family's schedule over a two-day period. Karen agreed, noting, "People seemed more comfortable and open in the house than they would have been at the mortuary. Also, I felt nurtured by people coming into our home offering warmth, support, and help."

CHAPTER 28

Creating a Personalized Funeral or Memorial Service

The difference between a funeral and a memorial service is that the body is present at a funeral. Because of this, funerals are generally held within a few days, but sometimes as much as a week after the death. The time frame is more flexible with a memorial service, as is the location.

It is comforting when many people care enough to come and pay their respects, but bigger is not always better. While I have officiated at many large funerals, the intimacy of a small group can sometimes be more comfortable and comforting than a large crowd. I've also found that people are more willing to open up and share at a small and informal gathering.

Because traditional religious services are available through clergy, I offer here three examples of alternative ceremonies. Elements from these, such as the candle rite in Sara's ceremony, could easily be incorporated into a traditional service.

Understanding the basic structure of a funeral or memorial service will make it easier for you to create a personally meaningful ceremony. Looking over the brief descriptions of each section below will provide a sense of the general flow of a ceremony. The samples that follow will further illustrate, as well as provide wording that you may want to use in the ceremony you create.

Structure of a Ceremony

OPENING WORDS

The first section of a ceremony draws people together, states the purpose of the gathering, and sets the tone. The following examples illustrate different levels of formality.

Traditional: Dearly beloved, we have gathered here to mourn the death of _____, and commend his soul to God.

Contemporary: We have come together to share our grief over the loss of _____, and to honor and celebrate what she brought to our lives.

Casual: We've come here to say goodbye to _____, and then to have a rip-roaring good time, because that's exactly what he would want!

A brief observation about the person's life brings those in attendance into connection with the character and spirit of the person being honored. An easy way to do this is to use a phrase that is typical of the person and captures the spirit of his or her personality. It might even be humorous if the family prefers to keep the occasion light. Choose something that not only provides a vivid and affectionate picture of the person, but also sets the desired tone.

The following are some examples:
We will all miss
~ being welcomed into her kitchen for a cup of tea.
~ hearing his novel thoughts on minimalism.
~ enjoying the beautiful flowers she grew
~ his terrible jokes and his sage advice
~ seeing the twinkle in her eyes when she was excited by something

INVOCATION

This section serves to invoke a higher power. For some, that is their God. For others, it is connecting with a spiritual state of mind and heart. This section also serves to invoke a sense of community.

Feeling connected to something greater than ourselves—be it God, spirit, nature, or friends and family—allows us to confront the loss with a sense of support.

The invocation should honor the beliefs of the deceased, while also being respectful of other points of view.

The following sentence is an example of how each person can be invited to enter into a prayerful state according to their own beliefs: *In the moment of silence that follows, you may offer a prayer, your gratitude, or a personal blessing.* The second sample ceremony provides an example of how to create community without invoking a higher power.

THOUGHTS ON LIFE AND DEATH

It is usually appropriate, often helpful and healing, to speak of our mortality in a way that provides perspective, and offers insights. In addition to religious passages, I often use quotes from secular sources, such as poems, passages from novels, and excerpts from essays. The "Resources" section offers suggestions for helping you find the right material to quote.

Like the Invocation, this section also needs to reflect the beliefs and values of the deceased, while being respectful of the beliefs of those most deeply impacted by the loss. On occasion, I have used this section to offer more than one way of looking at life and death, and then focusing on the common ground that different points of view share—even Buddhists and Baptists have some common ground. When there are a range of beliefs to be considered, you can include something from each tradition, or keep it spiritually inclusive.

This section of the ceremony may be philosophical and explored in some depth, or you may want to keep it brief, with perhaps even a touch of humor. I once recounted the story of a young man who was less than patient with metaphysical musings. After biding his time as others in a group discussed their thoughts, he finally burst forth and interjected, "It's not that complicated! When you get up there The Man says, 'Did you have a good time? Did you hurt anybody? Well, come on in then.' And that's all there is to it!" I then addressed the young man's life, using his perspective of what was important.

MUSIC AND READINGS

Music is often included in the ceremony, but isn't a requirement. You might want to use hymns, an appropriate popular song, a vocalist performing "Ave Maria," or a group sing of something like "Turn, Turn, Turn." There is a wonderful communal feeling evoked when everyone sings together. An instrumental piece that provides space for reflection can also be lovely.

"What A Wonderful World" is a popular choice for music and can be paired with a slideshow of photos of the deceased's life. Other musical suggestions can be found online, or perhaps in the music collection of the deceased.

Select music or readings that are not only appropriate for the occasion, but also appropriate for the individual. Readings can be a way for family members or friends to participate. An online search for "funeral poems" will provide a wide selection of possibilities.

CELEBRATING THE LIFE

Life overview: A format that works well is for the clergy person or officiant to provide an overview of the individual's life, highlighting important events and aspects. It might include family, career, setbacks and challenges, as well as triumphs. It's nice to include little known but insightful details that illustrate character and personality. The overview often provides a chronological framework for the tributes that will follow.

The life overview should be at least two paragraphs but usually no more than a page and a half. It often begins with birth date and location, but could begin with a formative incident, or key factors from his or her youth. While it doesn't have to be in chronological order, that is often the simplest way to organize this section. Ending with something about the nature of the individual's death and how he or she dealt with it is common, but one could end with an important event and highlight a memory that all present will want to carry forward in their mind when thinking of this person.

Tributes: It works well to have two or three designated people share their remembrances first, with each one focusing on a different aspect of the individual's life. Others are then invited to offer thoughts or tell stories.

Once the first speakers get the ball rolling, others will be a little more comfortable coming forward to share their thoughts and memories. I sometimes have a final person designated to speak to round out this section of the ceremony.

Occasionally, a speaker will talk for too long and sometimes it is necessary for the officiant to interrupt and gently point out that others also would like a chance to speak.

RITES

Symbolic action that addresses the loss is most helpful when it also reinforces what is not lost. The sample ceremonies offer examples that provide a symbolic way of saying goodbye, and also affirm what can never be lost.

You could ceremonially place personal mementos inside the casket before it is closed, saying something like, "While these items will go with Mary, there is much of her that will always be with us."

Planting a tree, or tossing flowers into a river can also be meaningful if you hold the ceremony outdoors.

There might be rituals in your religious or cultural heritage that would be appropriate, or with some adjustments would be fitting.

Looking over the person's life might provide inspiration for something unique and perfect for that individual.

CLOSING WORDS

This section of the ceremony often includes a prayer or poem offering comfort and hope, and can also include:

~ Thank you for coming.

~ Thank you for support.

~ The need for continuing support (along with guidance on how to do so.)

~ Information regarding what follows, such as burial at the cemetery or a reception.

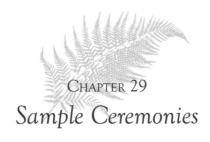

Chapter 29

Sample Ceremonies

*A*s you will see in the sample ceremonies, not every element is included, and sometimes there is an additional, brief section. The general structure and flow, though, is the same.

The first sample ceremony is short, simple, and informal. The second is an outdoor ceremony created for an agnostic gentleman. The third has a more traditional feel, and while not religious, is strongly spiritual.

Note to those performing a ceremony: Speak slowly, and pause at the end of every paragraph. Practice reading the ceremony aloud a number of times until you are comfortable with the text.

Please note that sections in italics in the sample ceremonies would need to be rewritten to reflect the individual being honored. Make other changes as necessary or desired.

Ceremony One: Simple and Casual

This first sample ceremony is a short ritual that utilizes only Opening Words, a slide show as Life Review, Tributes, and Closing Words.

Linda

We have gathered here this afternoon because Linda held a special place in our lives. *She had her own sense of the world, her own sense of style, and her very own way of relating a news story.*

We are here to bless her spirit, and we're here to invite her spirit to live on in the stories we tell. Linda's sons would love to hear stories of their mom—ones that are new to them, and one's where the story becomes richer or funnier with each retelling.

While we watch a montage of photos from her life, let yourself be reminded of the large and small stories of Linda's life; stories that illustrate her strengths and weaknesses (*her love of ice cream!*), her humor, and her perspective on life.

Tributes were offered by friends and family.

After allowing time for people to share their memories, close by saying:

We bless Linda for having been. We bless her spirit as it moves away from us. And we bless the spirit of Linda that will always live within our hearts.

On behalf of Linda's family, I thank all of you for coming today and sharing your stories. Thank you for the support you have provided to Linda and her sons over the last four months. I hope that you will all continue to offer stories and support, warm hugs, occasional tears, and much laughter.

Ceremony Two: Nontraditional and Secular

Chaz

OPENING WORDS

We have come together this afternoon to share grief over the loss of Charles MacRae, and also to honor and celebrate his life.

Chaz was a man with the capacity for great enjoyment, and the courage to pursue his dreams—he started his own business, he traveled to exotic locations, and he was always happy planning new projects here at the house and spending time with his family. Chaz had a most interesting life, and he lived it to the fullest.

All of you bring with you memories of your times with Chaz. A little later we'll take time to share some of those memories; the stories of joy and sorrow, of delightful, and even difficult times you shared with him. Like all of us, Chaz sometimes provoked frustration in those around him. He was human, and had his share of human failings. Without that humanness, though, there would not have been as much in his life to evoke the respect and admiration that made all of you so proud to have him as husband, father, brother, and wonderful friend.

It is because of your love and affection for Chaz that his death leaves such an empty place in your life. Adlai Stevenson said, "Our lives take their meaning from their interlacing with other lives, and when one life is ended those into which it was woven are also carried into darkness."

In our sorrow, we come together with others who also feel this sense of loss. Sharing the grief somehow makes it a little easier to bear.

INVOCATION

Chaz was not a religious man, and we want to respect his point of view. He did not believe in a higher spirit, but he had great faith in the human spirit. To honor that, we celebrate the beauty and strength of the human spirit that glows within us all.

In an exchange of fellowship, will you all please reach out to take the hand of the person on either side of you? Each one of us has our own connection to Chaz. And through Chaz, we are all connected to one another.

It is important that we periodically experience a strong sense of connection with community, particularly when we are shaken by the loss of someone we care about. Take a moment now to be fully aware of this feeling of deep connection with others.

Closing your eyes, slowly breathe in, and out, together. A breath in, and a breath out. As one, we breathe in; and as one we breathe out.

Gently squeeze hands to express this fellowship of spirit, sending the energy of love circling around and through this gathering.

I ask that you now focus this love on Chaz's family, offering your heart's blessings to them during this difficult time.

For all of us, but for Kathleen, Daniel, and Molly particularly:

We invite the power of love and grace to bring support through the pain and struggle of loss.

We invite the power of inner strength and peace.

We invite the healing power of gratitude—

for all that has been,

for all that is,

and all that will come to be.

We give thanks for Chaz's broad and generous spirit.

We give thanks for the varied ways we are able to offer
support to one another.

And most of all, we give thanks for the power of love,
knowing that it lives on in our hearts no matter
what happens.

Releasing hands, remember that we are all part of an infinite and unfathomable universe; and though we cannot measure exactly how, trust that the currents of love move us ever forward.

THOUGHTS ON LIFE AND DEATH

Like Chaz, Corliss Lamont believed in the power of the human spirit, and he explores it in this piece titled "Meditation."

"No philosophy or religion ever taught can prevent the wholly natural reaction of the human heart to grieve when there is loss. Yet we always remain grateful for his having lived and for our having know him in the full richness of his personality.

"Nothing now can detract from the joy and beauty that we shared with him; nothing can possibly affect the happiness and depth of experience that he himself knew. What has been, has been— forever. The past, with all its meanings, is sacred and secure. Our love for him and his love for us, cannot be altered by time or circumstance.

"We rejoice that he was and still is part of our lives. His influence endures in the unending consequences flowing from his character and deeds; it endures in our own acts and thoughts. We shall remember him as a living, vital presence. And that memory will bring refreshment to our hearts and strengthen us in times of trouble."

LIFE OVERVIEW

(Not included here in full, only the beginning and end.)

Today we honor Chaz through looking back on the important developments of his life. *Little Charlie was born in Madison, Wisconsin, in 1943, the second son of a dairy farmer. ...*

... Chaz's illness made his last months less than easy. Nonetheless, he reached out to engage in life, and to stay connected to those he held most dear. His last words were to say thank you to his wife and daughters. How lovely to have one's last lucid moments be brimming with gratitude.

In your sorrow at his passing, it is good to remember what it was in him that you want to live on within yourself.

You release him, yet you keep a part of him always:

the ways in which he touched your hearts,

the ways in which he influenced your thinking and
your approach to the world,

the ways in which he impacted on your path and your very
being will remain.

And so, pieces of him will live on, continuing to reverberate through each one of you.

CELEBRATING THE LIFE

Theodore Webb said, "When we remember a man, it is more than the man who is remembered. We remember what we are because of what he was; and what he was because of what we are."

We'd like now to share some memories and stories about Chaz. Several people have expressed a desire to speak, and then we'll open to others who would also like to share their thoughts and remembrances.

TRIBUTES
[Offered by friends and family. Then officiant says:"]

Chaz's life touched all of yours in some very special ways, and I encourage you to continue sharing your favorite memories of him—the moments that inspired affection and admiration, times that brought forth laughter or insight. These remembrances are precious, and serve as reminders that what Chaz brought to your lives, will remain with you always.

ROSEMARY RITE

Molly and her mom have created bouquets of rosemary, an herb long associated with remembrance. In the fire pit Chaz built many years ago, we lit a fire earlier today to symbolize the fire in the spirit of his personality. You are each invited to throw a bouquet of rosemary onto the fire and say aloud what you will always remember about Chaz.

[Molly goes first to demonstrate—"I will always remember your willingness to take on new adventures in life, and will do my best to let that live on in me. I thank you for . . . ." Officiant orchestrates bringing the others in. After everyone has had a turn, the officiant continues.]

The smell of rosemary, fresh or burning, is a sweet and lovely scent. So, too, is the fragrance of memory. May this sweetness provide solace when you are most in need of comfort.

CLOSING WORDS

Once again, please join hands. Let us close our eyes and slowly breathe together, holding one another in the light. This is a tradition of Quaker origin that holds great beauty and meaning in its simplicity: Gather in community and hold one another in the Light. So in this moment of silence, simply hold one another in the light. [A long pause.]

May your memories of Chaz, and your love and affection for him, live forever in such a place of illumination.

On behalf of Chaz's family, I thank all of you for coming here this afternoon, for sharing your memories, and for offering your support.

Ceremony Three: Traditional and Spiritual

Sara's Memorial

Small taper candles are handed to guests as they arrive. An eight-inch pillar candle sits on a table at the front, flanked by a photo of Sara and a simple vase of flowers. The officiant lights the candle to begin the ceremony.

OPENING WORDS

[Lighting the pillar candle on the front table, the officiant says:]

This candle is lit as a symbol of Sara's spirit.

We have come together this afternoon to mourn the death of Sara Thompson, and to share grief over the loss. We are here also to express our love, respect, and admiration as we celebrate her life.

(The following paragraph is provided as an example only. Write your own paragraph that describes the person you are honoring.)

Sara had an interesting and meaningful life, and we all have been a part of it. Some of you may have known her as a girl or young woman in the Midwest. Many of you met her after she moved to Arizona in her thirties, and some have only gotten to know her over the last several years. You've all heard stories about her life, and you'll hear more stories about her today. This is a time for honoring her life, and exploring how Sara used her accomplishments and struggles to enlarge her understanding of herself and the world. Mythology fascinated her—she loved the stories, the archetypes, and the way they led her into a deeper spiritual understanding. And she loved sharing on so many levels with all of you.

At Sara's request, please hug the person on either side of you, and let the spirit of Sara bless you with her warmth and support.

INVOCATION

There was a special radiance that came through Sara; an illuminated essence that was pure Sara, and yet whispered of something greater.

There is something of this divine essence within us all. We ask that the sacred source of that essence be present here today to bless this gathering with a spirit of healing.

Closing our eyes, let us connect with the divine source of love, which surrounds and suffuses us all. Allow the illuminating energy of this spirit to be felt in your heart.

May the divine source of love, source of all life, grace us with a heightened sense of the power and mystery of life, and of love. May we come to know that this great love extends beyond all boundaries.

May the love that illuminates all of our beings shine through each one of us and into the hearts of those whose lives are forever changed by this loss.

In the moment of silence that follows, you may offer a prayer, ask for comfort and guidance, or let your heart simply rest in the peace of stillness.

[After a moment]

We will all miss feeling Sara's words of support like a warm embrace, so offer your compassion to others as a tribute to Sara.

(Alternate Choice for Invocation)

Let us join together in a spirit of prayer.

God of loving radiance, creator of this earth and the heavens,
 who guides our spirits with love and wisdom,

we invite your presence to be felt in our midst.

Though your fuller wisdom is sometimes beyond our understanding, we do our best to trust in your love.

As we bring your sacred love into our hearts, we ask that there may be healing and comfort offered to all of those gathered here in sorrow.

We ask for your blessing on Sara, whom you gifted with the spark of life, and through that brought blessing to us all.

Help us to remember that love is greater than sorrow, and that love endures even through the great pain of loss.

We offer our gratitude for the gift of life, the great gift of love, and for all gifts of grace. Amen.

THOUGHTS ON LIFE AND DEATH

When someone we know and care for dies, the concept of mortality takes on a more palpable presence. It is fitting to speak of death today, and to reflect on it from Sara's point of view.

Sara believed, as do many of us here, that this lifetime is set within a larger context. We may have different ideas about the exact nature of that context, but from time immemorial, man has sensed there was something larger, something beyond this physical world. The prehistoric cultures that built Stonehenge, and painted on the walls of caves in France, left evidence they sensed there was something holy and sacred about life and what we do here on earth is somehow interconnected with realms beyond this.

A major difference between modern and ancient cultures is that their beliefs were based on a more direct experience of nature. The natural world, of which we are a part, shows us that just as life is followed by death, death is followed by rebirth. Day is followed by night, which leads to still another dawn. The seasons reiterate this cycle of rebirth—the coldest, darkest winter gives way, in time, to summer. The grain harvested in autumn becomes the seed of spring and grows again. Life and death are two aspects of one condition—the dark moon is but a passing phase of the bright moon.

Sara continues to exist. The essence of Sara Thompson is a part of God, the immortal source, creator of stars and spider webs—as are we all. Sara understood that when the body releases us through death, we move on through the cycles of existence. Death is not the last thing. It is no more than a cobweb that we brush through, a thin veil separating this existence from the next.

Sara's body is dead, but only her body. The spirit animated her body, and that did not perish when her body gave out. Even though the conditions of her existence have changed, her spirit has not ceased to be. Souls cannot be unmade. Her flesh has been transformed into ash, but her essence has now flowed on into other realms that you and I cannot truly even imagine.

READING

This poem by Robinson Jeffers offers us a glimpse of what he senses occurs when the spirit leaves the body.

I am not dead, I have only become inhuman:

That is to say,

Undressed myself of laughable prides and infirmities,

But not as a man

Undresses to creep into bed, but like an athlete

Stripping for the race.

The delicate ravel of nerves that made me a measurer

Of certain fictions

Called good and evil; that made me contract with pain

And expand with pleasure;
Fussily adjusted like a little electroscope:
That's gone, it is true;
(I never miss it; if the universe does,
How easily replaced!)
But all the rest is heightened, widened, set free.
I admired the beauty
While I was human. Now I am part of the beauty.
I wander in the air,
Being mostly gas and water, and flow in the ocean;
Touch you and Asia
At the same moment; have a hand in the sunrises
And the glow of this grass.
I left the light precipitate of ashes to earth
For a love-token.

THANK YOU

So many of you helped provide a circle of love and support for Sara. Her husband, Mike, and daughters, Marianne and Jenny, asked me to express their deep gratitude to those who cared for her in so many ways over a long period of time. Their gratitude for your many kindnesses—both large and small—will dwell forever in their hearts.

Those who offered such meaningful help may well feel that they were not the givers, but instead the receivers—to be witness to someone who bears life's difficulties with graceful honesty and strength is truly a privilege.

I'm sure that you all have many different memories of Sara's strength, of her intelligence, and her humor. A little later we'll have time for those who would like to come forward and share some of those memories with the rest of us.

First, though, I want to offer an overview of Sara's life.

LIFE OVERVIEW
(The text for Sara's overview is not included here.)

CELEBRATING THE LIFE

Like all of us, Sara was multifaceted, and family members and friends will remember her each in their own way. We'd like now to share some memories and stories about Sara—to reiterate her wisdom, to laugh at the humorous moments, and to remember the influence that she has had on our lives. Through this, may we remember to keep the best, most meaningful aspects of her alive within us. The first to speak is_____.

TRIBUTES
[Offered by family and friends]

Thank you for sharing your stories of Sara. These stories form a part of the legacy Sara leaves to her family and friends.

CANDLE RITE

In the midst of our sorrow, it is important we know that what Sara has brought to our lives will remain with us. She is interwoven into who we are. Pieces of her will live on, continuing to shine through each of us—*her daughters most of all. Marianne and Jenny carry not only her genes, but also her love, and her special light.*

Will the two of you please come forward.

[Music slowly comes up here if you want to use music during the candle lighting.]

Light your candles from Sara's flame in remembrance of the blessings of her spirit. Take her light as your own, and pass her light on.

[After lighting their candles from Sara's, the girls use their candles to light the candles of those sitting in the front row; then of all those sitting on the aisle, and those individuals pass the light on down the row. The girls then take their seats up front.]

Sara's light sparked something special in each one of us. She passed on the gifts of her spirit to all her family and friends. And her spirit, even still, can fill this room with light.

Allow her memory to fill your heart, as we join together in singing "I Will Remember You." Sara's dear friend Monique will lead us.

[As the last notes of the song fade out, officiant gently blows out Sara's candle.]
Though the flame of Sara's life is extinguished, her light will continue to illuminate our lives. We can keep that light burning within ourselves and allow her to shine through us.

Take a moment to meditate upon the light that she brought into your life . . . [A pause.]

Think about what it was in her that you would like to keep alive within yourself—

> Perhaps the warmth of her compassion,
> or her wry humor,
> her ability to add the right touch to something and
> make the ordinary quite special

Choose whatever it is that you want to live on within you.

Focus on that . . . see it shining in action . . . Now take that inside as yours, and consider it her parting gift to you.

Now, as we blow out our candles, we express gratitude for her many gifts, and we bless her spirit on its way. [Everyone blows out candles]

CLOSING WORDS

May the love illuminating all of our beings shine through each one of us and into the soul of Sara as she moves away from earthly life.

Let our gratitude shine upon her, filling her with the sweetness of earthly love.

May she be conscious of our love, we of hers.

May God's radiance shine upon her, filling her with the light of divine love.

May that radiance also shine upon and within us all. Amen.

On behalf of Sara's family, I'd like to thank all of you for coming today. Please join the family for a reception back at the house.

NOTES TO READER

I have often used this candle ritual in the daytime. Even with lights shining overhead and sun streaming through the windows, it was still very effective.

To avoid wax dripping, the unlit candle should be tilted into the lit candle, which remains upright.

The poem by Robinson Jeffers is "Inscription for a Gravestone."

Excerpts from *Druids*, an historical novel by Morgan Llywelyn, are included in the section, "Thoughts on Life and Death."

The song, "I Will Remember You," is by Sarah McLachlan. The lyrics were included in the handout so that people could sing along.

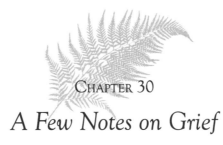

CHAPTER 30

A Few Notes on Grief

A century ago, there were clear guidelines as to how one behaved when faced with a loss, though the requisite behavior varied from one culture to another. In some cultures, one was required to be stoic and refrain from weeping in all but the most private circumstances. In other cultures, family members were expected to weep and wail quite openly, wear only black for at least a year, and were looked at askance if they didn't.

In contemporary Western culture, we are not hemmed in by such strict rules, but we have almost no guidelines to help us know how to behave or what to expect. Many grievers are unsure as to what is appropriate or even "normal." Most people expect to feel great sorrow, but are usually unprepared for the muddled mind and the overwhelming heaviness. Grieving loss is a natural response, and though it is among life's most painful experiences, it is important to remember that grieving helps us to heal.

I believe the following suggestions are especially important to be aware of in the early stages of loss.

1. Allow yourself to grieve in your own way, and in the time frame that feels right for you. Allow this of others as well. Also, be aware that it takes a few weeks for the initial shock

to wear off. Grief combined with shock can sometimes cause people to behave in ways that are not always easily understandable. Be patient with yourself, and others.

2. Take extra good care of yourself. If you have been the primary caregiver, you are likely exhausted on all levels. You will need time to restore not only your body, but also your spirit. Be very gentle with yourself: get plenty of rest, eat well, and drink lots of liquids—but go easy on the alcohol. And get some kind of exercise every day, even if it's only taking a walk around the block.

3. You needn't feel any rush to clean out the person's closet before you are ready to do so. Be careful about giving things away too soon, particularly in such a way that you could not get them back later if you change your mind. If you don't want the reminders around, box them up and store them for a while. I know one woman who gave several boxes to Goodwill, and then after a few months wanted some of the items back, but it was too late. Almost a year after giving some of my husband's things to family and friends, I suddenly wanted a particular item. Fortunately, I had given it to a dear friend of ours who was more than gracious about returning it.

4. If you can possibly do so, put off any important decisions for at least a year. In part, because there is only so much change we can handle at one time. The most cogent reason is that our minds generally are not working as well as we would like for quite a while, so sometimes we make decisions that don't serve us well in the long run. Not to mention that we are often overwhelmed by all of the feelings. Give yourself

as much time as you can to let the dust settle. Then sift through options and emotions before making important decisions.

5. It is important to have support after a major loss, and generally there are many gracious people who offer various kinds of support for a few weeks. When that extra support begins to evaporate, though, there may still be a need for it. If you can do so, ask for what you need. Also seek out other sources of support. Counseling is helpful for some people. Support groups can be very beneficial. About six months after Tony died, I found an on-line support group that was enormously helpful for me.

To find a local support group: do an online search for "grief support" plus the name of your geographical area. I tried a few different groups before finding one that felt right for me.

To find an on-line group: search for "grief support" plus "on-line groups." Look at several to discover what will best suit your needs. Some are open forums where individuals post their thoughts and feelings and others respond. GriefNet offers a number of groups that are targeted toward specific types of loss—loss of parent, child, or spouse, and has separate groups for children and teens who have suffered loss.

One advantage of GriefNet was being able to interact with others in my group whenever I wanted or needed to do so. When one member sends an e-mail message to the group, everyone receives a copy. No matter what time of day or night, there were usually at least a few people checking and responding to posts, so it felt like support and sharing were available 24/7. The groups are monitored by trained volunteers, and supervision is provided by a clinical psychologist.

Because it was a closed group, rather than a public forum, most individuals felt very comfortable sharing openly on GriefNet. With a limited number of participants in each group, a certain camaraderie and intimacy developed between those sharing tears and support. I found GriefNet to be a perfect place for me, but look at different sites to discover what will be a good fit for you.

Books

Books on grief can also lend support and guidance. There are many types of books that address grief, some are written by grief professionals, and others are mourners' journals. Read a few pages to see if the voice and the content feels comfortable and comforting to you.

GriefNet offers a categorized list of books on its site, and of course, online booksellers offer a wide range of books to choose from. Widownet.org offers a variety of resources, not solely for those who have been widowed.

There will be times when you may feel that you're crazy—or at least you're certain that some of the things you think and do are crazy. Most likely, you are not losing your mind, but you have lost someone you love very much. It helps to talk with others who are also grieving, or have been there, and will understand that grief has its own form of logic.

As deep as the pain can sometimes be, it will ease in time. You will never stop loving or missing your loved one. But eventually, and oh so gradually, the pain ebbs and you will figure out what you need to do with yourself in the next stage of your life.

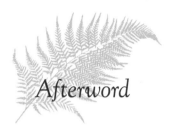

Afterword

*I*t was three o'clock in the morning when I walked down the hospital corridor away from the room where Tony had died. At some point before I reached the elevator, dazed, moving underwater, I realized, "My journey with Tony is now over."

Ten minutes later as I eased the nose of my car out of the parking structure, it struck me, "This is the beginning of my life without Tony."

In the middle of that dark December night, I didn't understand that my journey with Tony wasn't truly over, and never would be. Some time during the first few months after he died, I gradually realized that because so much of who Tony was had become interwoven with who I am, he would always be with me.

The road that stretched in front of me was difficult and painful in ways I could not have imagined, but my journey with Tony had developed within me a different kind of strength that helped me to live through even the days I didn't want to live through. Helping Tony to heal through his illness and live through his dying, together with all the love we shared, sustained me as I eventually moved into another place of meaning.

May all the lessons and love that you have shared sustain you wherever life and love, healing and dying, take you.

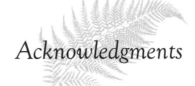

Acknowledgments

J will be forever grateful to those who offered support to Tony and me in so many meaningful ways during his illness. There isn't space to name everyone, but I want to acknowledge those who consistently went far above and beyond the call of duty throughout Tony's illness: Moray Greenfield and Robert Rigamonti, who provided a wealth of practical and emotional support to Tony and me for the entire twenty-two months; Corry Nethery and Loraine Shields who brought us delicious organic meals, week after week; Camille Ameen who graciously offered so much of her healing presence; and to our outstanding team of doctors, especially Dr. Roger Lerner, whose personal commitment made a world of difference to us. Tony and I were blessed.

I would like to thank Irene Borger, who inspired my writing and helped me find my voice as a writer; my dad, who encouraged me to be who I am, love life, and pursue what holds meaning; and my mother, who always reminds me to laugh, to trust, and to flow with life.

I am deeply grateful to all those who encouraged and supported me in this project over a period of many years. I want to specifically mention those who read various drafts, provided feedback, and kept me from drowning in words: Jennifer Ballentine for her early and continued interest and help; Devan Cook and my sister Chanelle Courtney for their valuable feedback, as well as their love and humor;

and Dixie Haas for her countless hours of patience, unflagging interest, and vast areas of knowledge.

I thank my editor, Maureen R. Michelson, who provoked me to clarify what I truly mean, helped shape the book, and served as midwife to its birth. Also, my thanks to Sherry Wachter for developing a graceful layout and a book cover better than I imagined. My special thanks to Ken Doka, who graciously offered to write the foreword. I am also grateful for the existence of Danton Press, and all who have contributed to the production of this book, including Candolin Cook, who provided her valuable perspective when I needed it.

Finally, I want to thank those who have included me in their journeys, and allowed me to share parts of their stories—for it is stories that help us heal and grow.

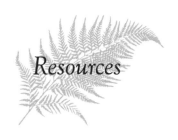

Resources

*D*irect links to the resources listed below can be found at my website: **www.healingthroughillness.com.**

I will continue to add additional links as I discover them. You may contact me via the Q&A section on my website with any additional questions, or if you have resource suggestions.

Patient Support

www.mealtrain.com helps friends and family more easily coordinate delivery of meals. It's free, includes a patient preferences section, and even sends out reminders.

www.patientslikeme.com offers connections to support for a wide range of medical conditions.

The following cancer-related sites offer information, articles, and a range of support. Many of these resources can be helpful for non-cancer patients also.

www.mercymedical.org provides long-distance charitable medical air transportation to and from specialized medical care.

www.cancercare.org provides free professional help to people with all cancers through counseling, education, as well as referral and direct financial assistance.

www.cancer.net is the American Society of Clinical Oncology's patient information website.

www.canceradvocacy.org National Coalition for Cancer Survivorship is the oldest survivor-led advocacy organization.

www.thewellnesscommunity.org has centers in most major cities with groups and classes where they provide free emotional support, education, and hope for people with cancer and their loved ones.

Caregiver Support

www.caregiver.org Family Caregiver Alliance offers newsletters, discussion groups, and articles on a wide variety of topics relating to caregiving. Check out their "New to Caregiving" section.

www.caringtoday.com Provides general caregiving advice, offers specific information for a range of diseases, can help you find the resources you need where you live, and offers financial and legal information.

www.strengthforcaring.com is an online resource and community for family caregivers.

www.archrespite.org National Respite Network and Resource Center provides information on why respite is important for caregivers, and how they can access outside resources.

www.caring.com has a focus on elder care, including resources for outside help, financial and legal matters, home care, caregiver support, and helpful suggestions for patients with Alzheimer's. Covers both general issues, such as caring for the caregiver and medical directives, as well as very specific topics such as what circumstances qualify a veterans widow for benefits.

Area Agency on Aging advocates, plans, coordinates, develops and delivers services for adults aged 60 years and older, persons of any age with HIV/AIDS, adults aged 18 years and older with disabilities and long-term care needs, and family caregivers. An online search will yield the nearest agency in your locale.

Advance Directives

The following websites provide valuable information to help with this difficult and important step.

www.caringinfo.org/PlanningAhead

www.respectingchoices.org

A booklet, *Hard Choices for Loving People*, is available on-line at **www. hardchoices.com.**

Talking About Death Won't Kill You, by Virginia Morris; Workman Publishing Co.

Body Donation

www.sciencecare.com accepts donations from every state in the U.S., except Minnesota and New Jersey. A highly reputable company, they cover all costs and logistics of transporting a body, and will even file a death certificate and return cremated remains to the family at no charge.

Ethical Will

www.mylifesgift.com offers ideas, introductory phrases, and provides a sample. There is also a template for creating a legal will. There are many websites that address ethical wills, some of which are quite good, but I like this site because it has depth, simplicity, and only minimal advertising.

Make A Wish

Most people have heard of the Make-A-Wish Foundation (**www.wish.org**) that grants wishes to children with a terminal illness. Foundations granting wishes to adults include:

www.dreamfoundation.com grants final wishes to terminally ill adults over the age of 18. (805) 564-2131

www.foreveryoungseniorwish.org reaches out to residents of nursing homes, assisted living facilities, hospice programs, home-bound individuals and adult day care facilities, regardless of age, to help make their dreams come true. (901) 299-7515

www.reelingandhealing.org hosts fly-fishing retreats for women and men with cancer. Also offers a retreat for family, friends and caregivers once each year. (866) 237-5725

www.secondwind.org A non-profit organization that grants wishes to older adults living in eldercare facilities or in hospice care. (678) 624-0500

Children

Resources for Adults
www.supersibs.org offers advice and resources to parents, teachers and others, to help them know how to support and comfort siblings of young patients.

www.hospicenet.org provides excellent advice on talking about death and helping children cope, as well as offering suggestions to appropriately involve children.

Talking About Death: A Dialogue Between Parent and Child, by Earl A. Grollman; Beacon Press. A guide for parents that features a read-along story and answers to questions that children may ask about death.

When a Parent Has Cancer: A Guide to Caring for Your Children, by Wendy S. Harpham, M.D.; William Morrow Paperbacks. Dr. Harpham is a mother, physician and cancer survivor who knows firsthand the challenges of supporting children while also struggling with serious illness. Included is *Becky and the Worry Cup*, an illustrated children's book that tells the story of a seven-year-old girl's experiences with her mother's cancer.

Resources for Children
www.supersibs.org has an area called "Sib Spot" that provides direct support to siblings of young patients.

www.teenslivingwithcancer.org is a terrific resource for teens, and their friends.

When Someone You Love Has Cancer: A Guide to Help Kids Cope (Elf-Help Books for Kids) by Alaric Lewis; One Caring Place. Ages 13 and under.

The Fall of Freddie the Leaf: A Story of Life for All Ages by Leo Buscaglia; published by Slack. Ages 4 and up.

The Next Place by Warren Hanson; Bantam. Ages 5 and up.

What's Heaven? by Maria Shriver; St. Martins Press. Ages 5 and up.

When Someone Has a Very Serious Illness, by Marge Heegaard; Woodland Press. Ages 9 and up.

When Someone Very Special Dies, by Marge Heegaard; Woodland Press. Ages 9 and up.

Alzheimer's Patients

Both of the following organizations provide education and support for dementia patients and their caregivers, and can help in finding additional resources.

www.alz.org Alzheimer's Association

www.nia.nih.gov/Alzheimers/ The National Institute on Aging

Learning to Speak Alzheimer's: A Groundbreaking Approach for Everyone Dealing with the Disease by Joanne Koenig Coste; Mariner Books.

Loving Someone Who Has Dementia: How to Find Hope While Coping with Stress and Grief by Pauline Boss, PhD; Jossey-Bass.

The 36-Hour Day: A Family Guide to Caring for People with Alzheimer Disease, Other Dementias amd Memory Loss in Later Life by Nancy L. Mace and Peter V. Rabins; Grand Central Life & Style.

Home-Centered After-Death Care

The following websites provide practical information, inspiration, and creative suggestions:

www.Finalpassages.org

www.lastthings.net

www.ehow.com/how_5510483_build-own-pine-box-casket.html

This article from the *New York Times* on home funerals is worth reading: **www.nytimes.com/2009/07/21/us/21funeral.html**

Funeral and Memorial Planning

www.thefuneralsite.com offers general information, and pricing overview. The library contains a wide range of information on everything from selecting poetry to scattering ashes over the Grand Canyon.

www.planningafuneral.com/music.aspx offers a list of music that might be suitable for inclusion in funerals.

Remembering Well, by Sarah York; Jossey-Bass. A beautiful guide to creating personalized ceremonies, includes text to use in the ceremony, and rituals.

Great Occasions, edited by Carl Seaburg; Skinner House Books. Contains a wide range of poetry and short readings for ceremonies.

In Memorium: A Guide to Modern Funeral and Memorial Services, by Edward Searl; Skinner House Books.

Grief

All of the following sites offer resources and information, as well as online support:

www.griefnet.org

www.widownet.org

www.growthhouse.org

List of Rituals

Index

About the Author

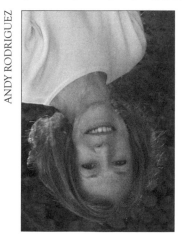

ANDY RODRIGUEZ

Candice Courtney's husband, Tony, died in December of 1998, three-and-a-half years after the death of her father. As a result of her own experiences, Ms. Courtney saw a need for support that brought greater meaning into the journey. She began working with individuals and families creating rituals to support them as they moved through the difficult, and usually foreign, passages of approaching death and grieving loss.

Ms. Courtney has an extensive background in the area of ritual. Since 1995, she has designed, written, and performed more than 200 ceremonies for life passages, including weddings, funerals, births, divorces, retirements, and milestone birthdays. She finds the rites associated with anniversaries and seasons, as well as life's everyday rituals, equally as intriguing as the major ceremonies. She has studied ritual in cultures worldwide and the essential role it has played throughout human history.

Ms. Courtney's professional presentations include organizations such as the National Hospice and Palliative Care Organization (NHPCO), Hospice and Palliative-Care Nurses Association (HPNA), and the Association for Death Education and Counseling (ADEC), of which she is a member. Her articles on coping with serious illness and grief have appeared in publications nationally. She also presents interactive workshops to help professionals include supportive ritual in the dying and bereavement processes.

Ms. Courtney is currently writing a book on rituals to support those mourning a loss. She can be reached through the publisher's web site: www.DantonPress.com